Feeding and nutrition
of infants and young children

Guidelines for the WHO European Region, with emphasis on the former Soviet countries

WHO Library Cataloguing in Publication Data

Feeding and nutrition of infants and young children : Guidelines for
the WHO European Region, with emphasis on the former Soviet
countries / Kim Fleischer Michaelsen...[et al.]

(WHO regional publications. European series ; No. 87)

1.Nutrition 2.Policy-making 3.Guidelines 4.Europe
I.Fleischer Michaelsen, Kim II.Series

ISBN 92 890 1354 0   (NLM Classification: QU 145)
ISSN 0378-2255

Text editing: Frank Theakston
Cover design: Sven Lund

World Health Organization
Regional Office for Europe
Copenhagen

Feeding and nutrition of infants and young children

Guidelines for the
WHO European Region,
with emphasis on the
former Soviet countries

Kim Fleischer Michaelsen, Lawrence Weaver,
Francesco Branca and Aileen Robertson

WHO Regional Publications, European Series, No. 87

ISBN 92 890 1354 0
ISSN 0378-2255

contents

Foreword .... *ix*

Acknowledgements xi

Recommendations xii

Introduction 1
  Why is this publication needed and for whom is it intended? 1
  Some determinants of health in Europe 3
  The contents of this book 4
  Terminology 5
  Adaptation and implementation of these guidelines 5
  References 7

1. Health and nutritional status and feeding practices 9
  Nutrition-related health problems in young children 9
  Feeding practices and recommendations 26
  References 35

2. Recommended nutrient intakes 39
  Introduction 39
  Recommendations are derived from requirements 40
  Nomenclature of recommended nutrient intakes 42
  References 43

3. Energy and macronutrients 45
  Energy 45
  Energy density 51
  Protein 54
  Fat 59
  Carbohydrates 62
  References 66

4. Vitamins 69
  Vitamin A 69
  B vitamins 73
  Vitamin C 74
  Vitamin D 76
  References 79
  Appendix 81

5. Minerals other than iron 85
   Iodine 85
   Zinc 91
   Calcium 93
   Sodium 94
   References 96
   Appendix 98

6. Control of iron deficiency 101
   Introduction 101
   Physiology and pathophysiology of iron 105
   Symptoms and consequences of iron deficiency 112
   Complementary foods and control of iron deficiency 114
   Other interventions to control iron deficiency 118
   References 122

7. Breastfeeding and alternatives 127
   The importance of breastfeeding 127
   Nutritional benefits of breastfeeding 127
   Non-nutritional benefits of breastfeeding 133
   Importance of maternal nutrition 139
   Practical aspects of breastfeeding 141
   How to increase the duration and incidence of breastfeeding 146
   Contraindications to breastfeeding 152
   Alternatives to breastfeeding 156
   References 161

8. Complementary feeding 169
   What is complementary feeding? 169
   Physiological development and maturation 170
   Why are complementary foods needed? 174
   When should complementary foods be introduced? 174
   Composition of complementary foods 177
   Practical recommendations for the introduction of
      complementary foods 181
   What are the best foods to prepare for infants? 184
   Some practical recommendations for food preparation 195
   References 196

9. Caring practices 199
   Introduction 199
   The UNICEF Care Initiative and nutrition 199

Factors affecting the ability of caregivers to carry out
    optimum feeding practices 202
Care for girls and women and the consequences 203
Feeding young children 204
Psychosocial care 208
Resources for care 209
References 214

10. Growth assessment 217
Introduction 217
How to measure growth and use growth charts 218
Reference populations 219
Interpretation of measurements of attained growth 222
Catch-up growth 224
References 224

11. Dental health.. 227
Prevalence of dental caries 227
How caries are formed 229
Relationship between diet and dental caries 229
Prevention of dental caries 230
References 232

12. Food safety 235
Introduction 235
Microbiological contamination 235
Chemical contamination 240
References 244

Annex 1. The International Code of Marketing of Breast-milk
          Substitutes and subsequent relevant resolutions of the
          World Health Assembly 247

Annex 2. Prevention of mother-to-child transmission of HIV 279

Annex 3. Infant feeding in Integrated Management of
          Childhood Illness 283

Foreword

A child's first 2 or 3 years of life are the most crucial for normal physical and mental development. Nevertheless, current feeding practices in some countries may be doing more harm than good to the development of young children. Children under 3 years of age are vulnerable to poor nutrition; the growth rate during this period is greater than at any other time, and there thus exists an increased risk of growth retardation. Also, the immunological system is not fully mature at this age, resulting in a risk of frequent and severe infections. Both cognitive and emotional potentials start to develop early, and so the foundations of intellectual, social and emotional competencies are also established during this period. In summary, poor nutrition during the early years leads to profound defects including delayed motor and cognitive development, behavioural problems, deficient social skills, a reduced attention span, learning deficiencies and lower educational achievement.

Infants, especially those who have a low birth weight or are otherwise vulnerable, are at high risk of morbidity and mortality during the first 2 years of life, especially after 6 months of age. In the period after birth most infants, even the most vulnerable, grow and develop normally if they are exclusively breastfed. If foods or drinks are introduced too early or are not given safely in the correct quantity at the optimum time, growth rates falter dramatically and can lead to growth retardation. By the time these children are 2 years old, many will be stunted. This is irreversible, and as adults they will remain small and be likely to have reduced mental and physical capacities. To reduce the high prevalence of stunting – common among vulnerable groups in the European Region – national feeding guidelines based on those given in this book should be implemented by health ministries. This will promote normal growth and development in the first 3 years of life, especially for the most vulnerable.

Nutrition-related health problems during the first 3 years of life lead to short- and long-term consequences, such as cardiovascular disease, that limit human potential within society. Improving infant and young child nutrition should thus be a priority, and be seen as an integral part of social and economic development. During times of economic crisis countries face difficult choices, so it is imperative to advocate social sector investments, notably nutrition policies for young children. Failing to ensure that young children receive optimum nutrition is counterproductive. Faced with limited resources, countries may decide to reduce general expenditure by limiting resources devoted to the development of young children. In the long run, however, failing to invest in the young will be more costly to the state and to society. Future mental and physical capacity will be compromised and, in addition, treating the resulting preventable diseases will be extremely costly. By placing emphasis on the first three years of life and developing comprehensive nutrition policies, countries can avert many preventable deaths, avoid irreversible mental damage, and preserve a child's priceless endowment of emotional, intellectual and moral qualities.

The 1997 edition of UNICEF's State of the world's children *states: "Approximately half the economic growth achieved by the United Kingdom and a number of Western Countries between 1790 and 1980 ... has been attributed to better nutrition and improved health and sanitation conditions, social investments made as much as a century earlier". The social and economic costs of poor nutrition are huge. For this reason, international investment banks agree that investing in nutrition makes sense: it reduces health care costs and the burden of chronic preventable diseases in adulthood, it improves social and economic development and it promotes learning and intellectual capacity. No economic analysis, however, can fully do justice to all the benefits of sustained mental, emotional and physical development in childhood.*

In general, the central role that nutrition and feeding practices play with regard to the health and development of young children is not sufficiently well understood by enough health professionals. Health professionals should be a source of correct and consistent information on nutrition. These guidelines have been produced to facilitate this and strengthen the role of the health sector. A large proportion of the health service budget is used to treat preventable nutrition-related disorders, costs that could be substantially reduced if these disorders were prevented. Implementing these guidelines will enable countries to develop their own national nutrition policies for infants and young children. In doing this, the health sector can carry out its role effectively within this crucially important area of public health. Children represent the future of a nation, and these guidelines have been produced with the intention that young children, especially the disadvantaged, will have a better future.

Marc Danzon
Regional Director
WHO Regional Office
  for Europe
Copenhagen, Denmark

John Donohue
Regional Director
CEE/CIS and the Baltics
UNICEF Office for Europe
Geneva, Switzerland

Acknowledgements

This publication was prepared by WHO's Nutrition Policy, Infant Feeding and Food Security programme at the Regional Office in collaboration with the United Nations Children's Fund (UNICEF). The authors would like especially to thank Rachel Elsom and Ellenor Mittendorfer, who carried out most of the background research and helped draft the manuscript.

The financial support provided by the Governments of the Netherlands and the United Kingdom is gratefully acknowledged. In this context we would especially like to thank Elly Leemhuis-de Regt and Jacob Waslander of the Netherlands for their interest and support. Many individuals contributed to this book, and in particular Dr Bruno de Benois (WHO), Professor François Delange (Belgium), Professor Patrice L. Engle (United States), Dr Marco Jermini (WHO), Dr Lida Lhotska (UNICEF), Dr Yasmine Motarjemi (WHO), Dr Elizabeth M. Poskitt (United Kingdom), Professor Andrew Rugg-Gunn (United Kingdom) and Dr Jovile Vingraité (Lithuania).

Special thanks are also due to the participants attending the UNICEF/WHO Regional Consultation on Prevention and Control of Iron Deficiency Anaemia in Women and Children, held in Geneva in February 1999, and to the following who contributed to individual sections or reviewed the draft text: Dr Carlo Agostoni (Italy), Ms Helen Armstrong (United States), Professor Zulfiqar Bhutta (Pakistan), Professor Ken Brown (United States), Dr Nancy Butte (United States), Dr Michel Chauliac (France), Professor Forrester Cockburn (United Kingdom), Professor Kathryn Dewey (United States), Dr Conor Doherty (United Kingdom), Dr Henrik Friis (Denmark), Dr Serge Hercberg (France), Professor Olle Hernell (Sweden), Professor Peter Howie (United Kingdom), Ms Sandra Huffman (United States), Ms Hind Khatib (UNICEF, Geneva), Dr Felicity Savage King (WHO headquarters, Geneva), Professor Berthold Koletzko (Germany), Ms Sandra Lang (United Kingdom), Dr Christian Mølgaard (Denmark), Dr Olga Netrebenko (Russian Federation), Ms Nancy Jo Peck (Switzerland), Dr John Reilly (United Kingdom), Ms Patti Rundall (United Kingdom), Dr Werner Schultink (UNICEF, New York), Dr Roger Shrimpton (UNICEF, New York), Dr Inga Thorsdóttir (Iceland), Dr Abdelmajid Tibouti (UNICEF, Geneva), Professor Brian Wharton (United Kingdom), Professor Susan Reynolds Whyte (Denmark), Dr Anthony Williams (United Kingdom) and Dr Charlotte Wright (United Kingdom).

Recommendations

INTRODUCTION

It is recommended that each country review, update, develop and implement national nutrition and feeding guidelines for infants and young children, based on the recommendations in this publication.

HEALTH AND NUTRITIONAL STATUS AND FEEDING PRACTICES

It is recommended that each country establish nutrition surveillance of infants and young children as an integral part of its health information system.

Breastfeeding practices, feeding patterns and the nutritional status of infants and young children should be monitored regularly to enable problems to be identified and strategies developed to prevent ill health and poor growth.

RECOMMENDED NUTRIENT INTAKES

Each country should use recommended nutrient intakes for infants and young children, based on international scientific evidence, as the foundation of its nutrition and feeding guidelines.

ENERGY AND MACRONUTRIENTS

Provision of adequate dietary energy is vital during the period of rapid growth in infancy and early childhood. Attention must be paid to feeding practices that maximize the intake of energy-dense foods without compromising micronutrient density.

An adequate protein intake with a balanced amino acid pattern is important for the growth and development of the infant and young child. If the child receives a varied diet, however, protein quantity and quality are seldom a problem. It is prudent to avoid a high-protein diet because this can have adverse effects.

During complementary feeding and at least until 2 years of age, a child's diet should not be too low (because this may diminish energy intake) or too high in fat (because this may reduce micronutrient density). A fat intake providing around 30–40% of total energy is thought to be prudent.

Consumption of added sugars should be limited to about 10% of total energy, because a high intake may compromise micronutrient status.

VITAMINS

In countries where there is a high prevalence of childhood infectious disease, it is important to determine whether vitamin A deficiency is a public health problem.

In countries where rickets is a public health problem, all infants should receive a vitamin D supplement as well as adequate exposure to sunlight.

MINERALS OTHER THAN IRON

In countries where iodine deficiency is a public health problem, legislation on universal salt iodization should be adopted and enforced.

CONTROL OF IRON DEFICIENCY

Iron deficiency in infants and young children is widespread and has serious consequences for child health. Prevention of iron deficiency should therefore be given high priority.

When complementary foods are introduced at about 6 months of age, it is important that iron-rich foods such as liver, meat, fish and pulses or iron-fortified complementary foods are included.

The too-early introduction of unmodified cow's milk and milk products is an important nutritional risk factor for the development of iron deficiency anaemia. Unmodified cow's milk should not therefore be introduced as a drink until the age of 9 months and thereafter can be increased gradually.

Because of their inhibitory effect on iron absorption, all types of tea (black, green and herbal) and coffee should be avoided until 24 months of age. After this age, tea should be avoided at mealtimes.

Optimal iron stores at birth are important for the prevention of iron deficiency in the infant and young child. To help ensure good infant iron stores, the mother should eat an iron-rich diet during pregnancy.

At birth the umbilical cord should not be clamped and ligated until it stops pulsating.

BREASTFEEDING AND ALTERNATIVES

All infants should be exclusively breastfed from birth to about 6 months of age, and at least for the first 4 months of life.

Breastfeeding should preferably continue beyond the first year of life, and in populations with high rates of infection continued breastfeeding throughout the second year and longer is likely to benefit the infant.

Each country should support, protect and promote breastfeeding by achieving the four targets outlined in the Innocenti Declaration: appointment of an appropriate national breastfeeding coordinator; universal practice of the Baby Friendly Hospital Initiative; implementation of the International Code of Marketing of Breast-milk Substitutes and subsequent relevant resolutions of the World Health Assembly; and legislation to protect the breastfeeding rights of working women.

COMPLEMENTARY FEEDING

Timely introduction of appropriate complementary foods promotes good health, nutritional status and growth of infants and young children during a period of rapid growth, and should be a high priority for public health.

Throughout the period of complementary feeding, breast-milk should continue to be the main type of milk consumed by the infant.

Complementary foods should be introduced at about 6 months of age. Some infants may need complementary foods earlier, but not before 4 months of age.

Unmodified cow's milk should not be used as a drink before the age of 9 months, but can be used in small quantities in the preparation of complementary foods from 6–9 months of age. From 9–12 months, cow's milk can be gradually introduced into the infant's diet as a drink.

Complementary foods with a low energy density can limit energy intake, and the average energy density should not usually be less than 4.2 kJ (1 kcal)/g. This energy density depends on meal frequency and can be lower if meals are offered often. Low-fat milks should not be given before the age of about 2 years.

Complementary feeding should be a process of introducing foods with an increasing variety of texture, flavour, aroma and appearance, while maintaining breastfeeding.

Highly salted foods should not be given during the complementary feeding period, nor should salt be added to food during this period.

CARING PRACTICES

Policy-makers and health professionals should recognize the need to support caregivers, and the fact that caring practices and resources for care are fundamental determinants of good nutrition and feeding and thereby of child health and development.

GROWTH ASSESSMENT

Regular growth monitoring is an important tool for assessing the nutritional status of infants and young children and should be an integral part of the child health care system.

DENTAL HEALTH

It is recommended that the frequent intake of foods high in sugar, sugary drinks, sweets and refined sugar should be limited to improve dental health.

Teeth should be cleaned gently twice a day as soon as they appear.

An optimal fluoride intake should be secured through water fluoridation, fluoride supplements or the use of fluoride toothpaste.

FOOD SAFETY

Safe food, clean water and good hygiene are essential to prevent diarrhoea and food- and water-borne diseases, which are a major cause of poor nutrition, stunting and recurrent illness.

Breastfeeding should be encouraged even where contamination of breast-milk is a concern, and mothers should be reassured that the risk from contamination is very small compared with the overall benefits of breastfeeding.

Introduction

It is recommended that each country review, update, develop and implement national nutrition and feeding guidelines for infants and young children, based on the recommendations in this publication.

WHY IS THIS PUBLICATION NEEDED AND FOR WHOM IS IT INTENDED?

Optimum nutrition and good feeding of infants and young children are among the most important determinants of their health, growth and development. Good feeding practices will prevent malnutrition and early growth retardation, which is common in some parts of the WHO European Region. Poorly fed children have greater rates and severity of enteric and other infections, and they are at risk of dying prematurely. There is evidence to suggest that infant nutrition has long-term health consequences and plays a role in preventing the development of some chronic noncommunicable diseases in adults. Furthermore, micronutrient deficiencies, especially of iron and iodine, are associated with delayed psychomotor development and impaired cognitive function. Thus improvements in nutrition are desirable not only for the physical health and growth of young children but also for reducing the risk of infection, maximizing psychomotor development and school performance and, in the long term, improving opportunities for participating in social development.

The transition from an exclusively milk diet to one in which an increasing variety of foods is required to satisfy nutritional needs is a particularly vulnerable time. Poor nutrition and less-than-optimum feeding practices during this critical period may increase the risk of faltering growth and nutritional deficiencies. Despite the importance of infant and young child nutrition and feeding practices, limited attention has been paid to the need for guidelines based on scientific evidence. Recommendations on infant nutrition and feeding practices in the eastern part of the European Region are based on former Soviet recommendations, which are outdated and require revision. Moreover, a number of traditional dietary practices in the Region appear to have adverse effects on nutritional status; this is particularly true in the case of iron.

This publication has been produced to address this situation. It contains the scientific rationale for the development of national nutrition and feeding recommendations from birth to the age of 3 years, and is designed to provide information that will help national experts to develop or update their current national feeding recommendations.

This publication builds on WHO/UNICEF recommendations (1) and several national publications (2–6). In addition, a review of the literature has been carried out to develop appropriate scientifically based recommendations for Europe. In some key areas scientific evidence is limited, however, and it has therefore been necessary to base recommendations on pragmatic information, erring on the side of caution. Nevertheless, new data are continually becoming available, and it will be important to review the guidelines frequently and regularly.

The guidelines are designed for the WHO European Region, with emphasis on the countries that resulted from the dissolution of the former Soviet Union. Nutrition and feeding practices vary throughout the Region and these recommendations should be applied flexibly and be adapted to local and national needs and circumstances. Despite the wide range of socioeconomic conditions found between and within the Member States of the Region, it is believed that many recommendations can be applied universally. They are especially applicable to the most vulnerable groups of infants and young children living in deprived conditions. These are mainly found in the eastern part of the Region, but are also common in ethnic minorities and children of low-income families in western Europe.

This publication is primarily intended for ministries of health, paediatricians, dietitians, nutrition scientists and public health and other health professionals interested in nutrition who are concerned with the health of young children. It will allow policy-makers and national experts to develop or update their current national nutrition and feeding recommendations. It can also be used as a text for postgraduate education in child health. It is therefore hoped that the information provided will be effectively disseminated to these health professionals and to others working in relevant areas of the civil service and the private sector. There is now evidence to support claims that optimum infant and young child feeding will reduce the risk of some of the most prevalent adult diseases, such as cardiovascular disease, in the European Region. These guidelines, if implemented, will therefore not only have a positive impact on the health, growth and development of young children, but also strengthen their chances of growing up to be healthy adults.

SOME DETERMINANTS OF HEALTH IN EUROPE

Historically, life expectancy in the European Region has been high and is increasing. Since the dissolution of the Soviet Union, however, there has been a dramatic decrease in life expectancy at birth in those countries that were formerly part of it. Thus, in 1994, the average life expectancy in these countries was 66 years, which approaches that of developing countries (62 years). This decline in life expectancy is due in part to a rise in mortality among infants and young children.

Reducing premature mortality and so improving life expectancy can be achieved by improving the nutritional status of young children and their mothers. Although the nutrition of mothers is not dealt with in depth in this book, it is recognized that an optimum maternal diet will help to ensure the birth of healthy infants and improve their life expectancy. There is a sizeable body of evidence to suggest that good maternal nutrition supports optimal fetal development, which has long-term health consequences and plays a role in preventing the development of noncommunicable diseases, notably coronary heart disease, hypertension, stroke, chronic bronchitis, obesity and diabetes *(7–9)*. The mother's diet immediately prior to conception and during pregnancy influences the growth and development of the embryo and fetus. Where poor maternal nutrition is common (often linked to poverty) it is associated with low birth weight (< 2500 g), premature birth and high perinatal mortality, as well as the development of noncommunicable diseases in adulthood. The influence of early nutrition on cognitive development and adult health is another area of growing interest, particularly with respect to pre-term and low-birth-weight infants *(10–13)*. Investment in child nutrition will also contribute to a country's economic development *(11)*.

Poor child care is often associated with bad environmental conditions and poverty. While the impact of poverty is greatest in the eastern part of the Region, there is evidence of growing inequalities in western Europe *(14)*. The gap between rich and poor is widening in some countries. It is estimated that almost one third of children in the United Kingdom are living in poverty – three times the number in 1979 – and one in five lives in a household where nobody works – twice the rate of 1979 *(15)*. At the 1998 World Health Assembly it was pointed out that 32% of the population of the WHO European Region is living in poverty (the same percentage as found in developing countries). These statistics are derived from the global reports of the United Nations Development Programme (UNDP) *(16)* and UNICEF *(17)* and they illustrate the extent to which underlying poverty could predispose to malnutrition through a poor-quality diet.

Despite the high prevalence of poverty, there is little evidence of widespread protein-energy malnutrition (PEM) throughout the Region. Only in some of the central Asian republics are there signs of wasting and PEM. In Tajikistan and Uzbekistan, around 10% of children have been classified as suffering from PEM. However, in all of the central Asian republics and Azerbaijan, levels of growth retardation and stunting are high. In addition, levels of anaemia are high: 60% and 70% in Kazakhstan and Azerbaijan, respectively (see Chapter 1).

THE CONTENTS OF THIS BOOK

Chapter 1 reviews what is known about the current situation of child nutrition, together with limited information about current infant and young child feeding practices from selected countries in the Region.

Chapters 2–6 deal with nutrient recommendations, energy and the macronutrients (protein, fat and carbohydrates) and the most important vitamins and minerals. International recommendations on nutrient intake currently used by the European Union, the United Kingdom, the United States and WHO are compared. These recommendations provide a standard against which the adequacy of the diet of a population of infants and young children can be assessed. The difference between nutrient "requirements" and "recommendations" is explained, and how the latter concept has evolved and is designed to cover the wide range of individual variation in nutritional needs found within a population. The nutrient recommendations provide guidance on how much of each nutrient is required for the optimum health of young children, whether prevention of deficiency is enough, and whether overconsumption of a nutrient can be harmful. Other factors that affect the definition of nutrient recommendations, such as nutrient bioavailability, are also discussed. Iron deficiency anaemia is one of the major health problems throughout the Region and one that this publication aims to prevent, and therefore an entire chapter (Chapter 6) is devoted to this subject.

In Chapters 7–9, the importance of breastfeeding and the appropriate age for the introduction of complementary foods and fluids are reviewed. International experts agree that *exclusive* breastfeeding during early infancy is the most beneficial. The precise age at which appropriate, adapted family foods should be introduced will differ from infant to infant. Too early an introduction of complementary foods and fluids increases the risk of infection and reduces the benefit of exclusive breastfeeding. Too late an introduction can result in interruption of growth, undernutrition and an increased risk of illness. Chapter 9 is dedicated to the important role of the caregiver, and emphasizes that how infants and children are cared for can have a dramatic impact on their growth and development.

Chapter 10 deals with normal growth and development. Dental health, a major problem in children, especially in eastern Europe, is addressed in Chapter 11. Finally, Chapter 12 stresses the critical importance of preparing food for infants and children in a clean and hygienic way in the home. Poor food hygiene results in an increased incidence of diarrhoea, one of the main causes of growth retardation and stunting in the Region.

TERMINOLOGY

The term *exclusive breastfeeding* is frequently used in this book and means that all fluid, energy and nutrient requirements are provided by breast-milk alone, even in hot climates. The only possible exception is the addition of small amounts of medicinal supplements.

When foods are specifically prepared to meet the particular nutritional or physiological needs of the infant, they are described as complementary foods and could either be *transitional foods* or *adapted family foods*. These terms are used in the way that the term "weaning foods" is or was used. The term "weaning" is no longer recommended because, although it is derived from the old English wenian, meaning "to accustom", it has come to imply the cessation of breastfeeding. In this publication the term "weaning" is purposely avoided and it is stressed that the introduction of complementary foods should neither displace breast-milk nor initiate the withdrawal of breastfeeding.

The introduction of complementary foods in relation to the age of the child is shown in Fig. 1. Part A illustrates the contribution of breast-milk and other foods to total energy intakes at different ages; part B presents the same information as a percentage of total energy intake.

ADAPTATION AND IMPLEMENTATION OF THESE GUIDELINES

The foods that constitute the customary diet of infants in the WHO European Region are extremely varied because of the diversity of what is available and of cultural habits. To address these issues effectively it will be necessary for health ministries to produce national guidelines suited to the local situation. Before such guidelines can be developed, however, local

Fig. 1. Contribution of different food sources to young children's energy intake in relation to age

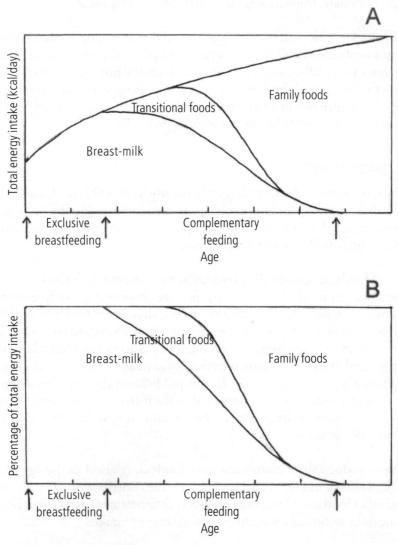

Source: World Health Organization (1).

conditions should be assessed. Gathering quantitative food intake data on the customary diet of young children is a challenge, but it is important to collect such information in addition to anthropometric data on weight and length. It is strongly recommended that health ministries, ideally jointly with ministries responsible for food and agriculture, undertake regular monitoring of the health and growth of infants and young children and that the process becomes an integral part of the national health and nutrition information system.

The recommendations presented in this publication will help health professionals involved in the care of infants and young children, and will assist policy-makers to develop national nutrition and feeding guidelines to prevent disease and achieve better health and development of young children. The health benefits are likely to persist into adulthood, and provide the foundation of a healthy start in life. These guidelines present a scientific consensus for health promotion and information to develop national recommendations. They provide a clear direction for the sustainable development of health and socioeconomic policy, and can help policy-makers identify resources needed to improve the health of young children and thus that of the population in future generations.

REFERENCES

1. *Complementary feeding of young children in developing countries: a review of current scientific knowledge.* Geneva, World Health Organization, 1998 (document WHO/NUT/98.1).
2. DEPARTMENT OF HEALTH, UNITED KINGDOM. *Weaning and the weaning diet. Report of the Working Group on the Weaning Diet of the Committee on Medical Aspects of Food Policy.* London, H.M. Stationery Office, 1994 (Report on Health and Social Subjects, No. 45).
3. CANADIAN PEDIATRIC SOCIETY, DIETITIANS OF CANADA & HEALTH CANADA. *Nutrition for healthy term infants.* Ottawa, Minister of Public Works and Government Services, 1998.
4. *Recommendations for the nutrition of infants: recommendations for health personnel.* Copenhagen, National Board of Health, 1998.
5. FOMON, S.J. Protein. *In:* Fomon, S.J. *Nutrition of normal infants.* St Louis, MO, Mosby, 1993, pp. 121–139.
6. GARROW, J.S. ET AL., ED. *Human nutrition and dietetics*, 10th ed. London, Churchill Livingstone, 1999.
7. BARKER, D.J.P., ED. *Fetal and infant origins of adult disease.* London, British Medical Journal, 1992.
8. OZANNE, S.E. & HALES, C.N. The long-term consequences of intrauterine protein malnutrition for glucose metabolism. *Proceedings of the Nutrition Society*, **58**: 615–619 (1999).
9. HERNANDEZ-DIAZ, S. ET AL. Association of maternal short stature with stunting in Mexican children: common genes vs common environment. *European journal of clinical nutrition*, **53**: 938–945 (1999).

8

10. Martorell, R. The nature of child malnutrition and its long term implications. *Food and nutrition bulletin*, **20**: 288–292 (1999).
11. Heaver, R. & Hunt, J.M. *Improving early childhood development – an integrated program for the Philippines*. Washington, DC, World Bank, 1995.
12. Gunnel, D. et al. Separating *in utero* and postnatal influences on later disease. *Lancet*, **254**: 1506–1507 (1999).
13. Lucas, A. et al. Fetal origins of adult disease – the hypothesis revisited. *British medical journal*, **319**: 245–249 (1999).
14. Daly, A. et al. Diet and disadvantage: observations on infant feeding from an inner city. *Journal of human nutrition and dietetics*, **11**: 381–389 (1998).
15. Department of Social Security, United Kingdom. *Opportunity for all: tackling poverty and social exclusion*. London, Stationery Office, 1999.
16. United Nations Development Programme. *Human development report 1997*. New York, Oxford University Press, 1997.
17. United Nations Children's Fund. *The state of the world's children 1998*. Oxford, Oxford University Press, 1998.

Health and nutritional status and feeding practices

It is recommended that each country establish nutrition surveillance of infants and young children as an integral part of its health information system.

Breastfeeding practices, feeding patterns and the nutritional status of infants and young children should be monitored regularly to enable problems to be identified and strategies developed to prevent ill health and poor growth.

NUTRITION-RELATED HEALTH PROBLEMS IN YOUNG CHILDREN

In order to develop national feeding guidelines and nutritional recommendations, sound data should be available on growth, nutrition-related diseases and feeding practices. The greatest concern is child survival, so mortality is one of the most important indicators of child health. The infant mortality rate is calculated as the number of deaths among children under 1 year of age divided by the total number of live births occurring in the same period. The under-5 mortality rate is calculated as the number of deaths among children under 5 years of age divided by the total number of live births occurring in the same period. Mortality data are usually reported routinely, but they may not be accurate in many countries because of poor or incomplete death certification.

Post-neonatal mortality (deaths among infants aged between 1 month and 12 months) is used as an indicator of poor living conditions and thereby poor nutrition, because many deaths during the first month of life are caused by congenital malformations and neonatal complications unrelated to nutrition. High mortality rates may not always be related to poor nutrition, and it is not always possible to establish a direct causal link between malnutrition and mortality. Nevertheless, a correlation has been demonstrated in several studies, and according to Pelletier *(1)* the relationship is continuous. Thus even mild and moderate malnutrition carries an increased risk of mortality.

Indicators of poor nutritional status can provide an early indication that a child is at risk (see Chapter 10). The most widely used are anthropometric.

For example, in children below the age of 5 years, measured weight and height can be compared with the weights and heights of children of the same age in a healthy reference population. The reference population recommended by WHO is that drawn up by WHO and the Centers for Disease Control and Prevention in Atlanta (CDC) *(2)*. Indices are usually expressed as standard deviations from the mean (Z score), centiles or percentage of the median.

The weight-for-height index is a measure of fatness or thinness and is sensitive to sudden changes in energy balance. A weight-for-height index more than two standard deviations below the mean is called "wasting" and indicates severe weight loss, which is often due to acute starvation and/or severe disease. Provided there is no serious food shortage, the population prevalence of wasting is usually below 5% even in poor countries. Children with a weight-for-height index more than two standard deviations above the mean are defined as overweight or obese.

Height-for-age is an index of the growth and development of the skeleton. A low value may be an expression of long-term exposure to nutritional inadequacy and indicate chronic malnutrition in children lacking essential nutrients, but it is also related to poor sanitary conditions, repeated infections, diarrhoea and inadequate care. Stunting is defined as a height-for-age index more than two standard deviations below the mean of the WHO/ CDC reference population. Stunting, unlike wasting, is relatively common throughout the European Region, especially in low-income groups.

The distribution of weights in the reference population used in the former Soviet Union is shifted to the right compared with that of the WHO/CDC population, so that the 5th centile of the Soviet reference corresponds approximately to the 10th centile of the WHO/CDC reference. This leads to a 5% overestimation of the prevalence of malnutrition and a 5% underestimation of the prevalence of obesity in countries that base their data on the former Soviet reference population.

Biochemical indicators are sometimes useful for assessing nutritional status, and some may provide an early indication of a specific nutrient deficiency, but because of their cost and invasiveness they cannot be measured routinely. Haemoglobin is one exception, because simple and relatively inexpensive field measurement methods have been developed. However, different haemoblobin cut-off points have been used to define mild and moderate anaemia *(3)*, and comparisons between countries are not always possible unless the same cut-off points have been used or the raw data are available.

It is often not possible to assess nutrient intake because food intake surveys are lacking. Moreover, data on breastfeeding rates from different countries cannot be compared easily because the definitions used are often different. Most surveys do not include data on exclusive breastfeeding. There is a need to stress the importance of exclusive breastfeeding for optimum child health (see Chapter 7) and create awareness of the need to measure its prevalence in every country. It is recommended that a standardized questionnaire for collecting data on breastfeeding and infant and young child feeding practices be developed for the WHO European Region to strengthen the current surveillance systems, which are not well established in most countries.

This chapter provides an overview of the situation in the European Region using the limited data available. For the purpose of comparison, the Member States of the WHO European Region have been divided into eight geographical regions, as shown in Table 1. Where possible, data from the central Asian republics (CAR) and the other members of the Commonwealth of Independent States (CIS) have been compared with those from western or southern Europe or from the Nordic countries. It is hoped that this comparison will highlight the disparity in health and nutritional status across the Region, and help to identify the nutritional problems of greatest concern. Based on the limited data available, some of the differences in infant and young child feeding practices are highlighted.

Mortality

Fig. 2 shows the wide disparity in infant and under-5 mortality rates in the European Region, ranging from the highest in CAR, particularly Tajikistan and Turkmenistan (over 55 and 75 per thousand live births for infant and under-5 mortality, respectively) to the lowest in the Nordic countries such as Finland and Sweden (5 per 1000 live births for both). The mortality rates in central and eastern Europe and in the Balkans fall between these two extremes at around 10–20 per 1000 live births. The difference between infant and under-5 mortality is relatively large in countries with high mortality rates. In contrast it is almost zero in Finland and Sweden, indicating that very few deaths occur after the first year.

Since the 1970s, infant mortality rates have been steadily decreasing across the Region (Fig. 3). However, while the averages for the European Union and the Nordic countries have dropped from 22 and 13 deaths per 1000 live births, respectively, in 1970 to just 5 in 1995, the figures for CIS and especially CAR remain significantly higher than in the rest of the Region.

Table 1. The Member States of the WHO European Region

Balkan countries	Baltic countries	Central Asian republics (CAR)	Central and eastern Europe	Commonwealth of Independent States (excluding CAR)	Nordic countries	Southern Europe	Western Europe
Albania	Estonia	Kazakhstan	Bulgaria	Armenia	Denmark	Andorra	Austria
Bosnia and Herzegovina	Latvia	Kyrgyzstan	Czech Republic	Azerbaijan	Finland	Greece	Belgium
Croatia	Lithuania	Tajikistan	Hungary	Belarus	Iceland	Israel	France
Slovenia		Turkmenistan	Poland	Georgia	Norway	Italy	Germany
The former Yugoslav Republic of Macedonia		Uzbekistan	Romania	Republic of Moldova	Sweden	Malta	Ireland
Yugoslavia			Slovakia	Russian Federation		Monaco	Luxembourg
				Ukraine		Portugal	Netherlands
						San Marino	Switzerland
						Spain	United Kingdom
						Turkey	

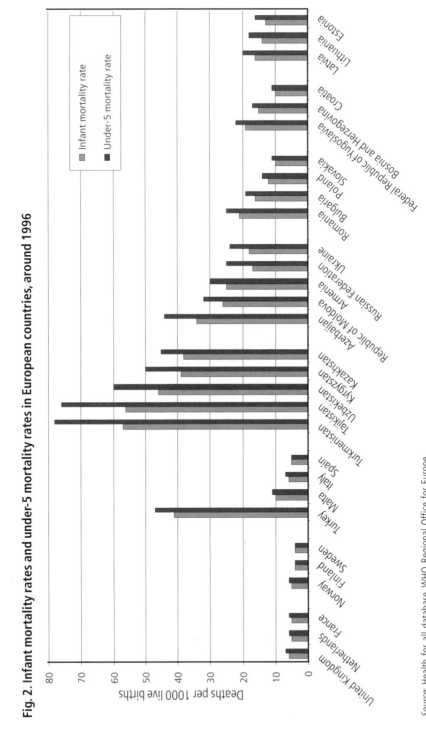

Fig. 2. Infant mortality rates and under-5 mortality rates in European countries, around 1996

Source: Health for all database, WHO Regional Office for Europe.

Fig. 3. Infant mortality rates in the European Region, 1970–1997

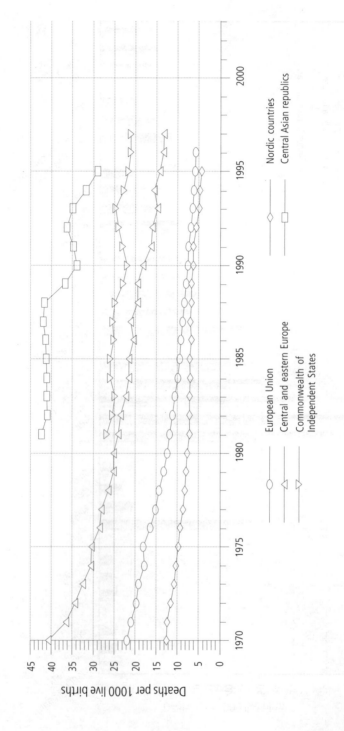

Source: Health for all database, WHO Regional Office for Europe.

Whereas in western European countries the primary causes of infant mortality are congenital malformations, injuries and "cot deaths" (sudden infant death syndrome), such deaths in countries with high mortality rates are mainly caused by infectious diseases. Poor nutritional status compromises the immune function of young children and makes them more susceptible to infections, particularly those affecting the respiratory and gastrointestinal tracts. In Azerbaijan, for example, the under-5 mortality rate from respiratory diseases is 24.5 per 1000 live births, while in Slovakia it is only 1.5 per 1000 live births.[1] In CAR, infants suffer from acute respiratory infections, diarrhoeal diseases and vaccine-preventable diseases such as tuberculosis; seven out of ten deaths are due to these illnesses, often in combination. Among children under 5, acute respiratory infections (notably pneumonia) are responsible for between 30% and 50% of all infant deaths. In Bulgaria and the Federal Republic of Yugoslavia, respiratory diseases are also the main cause of death in children (4).

Fetal, infant and child growth

Low birth weight

Low birth weight is defined as a birth weight of less than 2500 g. It is the result of either preterm delivery or intrauterine growth retardation, which can be related to poor nutritional status of the mother. Fig. 4 illustrates the prevalence of low birth weight across the European Region. Rather surprisingly, only Romania and the former Yugoslav Republic of Macedonia show a significantly higher prevalence (11%) compared with the countries of western Europe. Bulgaria and Poland, for example, both have a lower prevalence (6% and 5%, respectively) than the United Kingdom (7%).[1] Within the European Union, the proportion of low-birth-weight children has remained relatively constant over the past 20 years. Only the Nordic countries have seen a fall in the percentage of low-birth-weight infants.

In contrast, there appears to have been an increase in prevalence in CIS. In Armenia, for example, preterm delivery was recorded in 5.6% of live births in 1991 and this increased to 6.6% in 1996 (5). Births do not always take place in hospital, however, and so the information is not always complete. Furthermore, figures from eastern Europe may be biased by differences in reporting and in the definition of low birth weight. In some countries infants with a birth weight of less than 1000 g are not included because their risk of dying is so high. As a result, it is difficult to determine to what extent

---

[1] Data from the health for all database, WHO Regional Office for Europe.

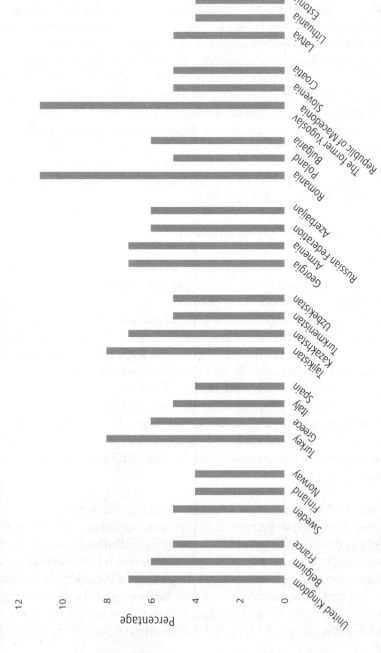

Fig. 4. Prevalence of low birth weight (< 2500 g) in Europe, 1990–1997

Source: Health for all database, WHO Regional Office for Europe.

the present data reflect the real situation. There is clearly a need to standardize the definition and collection of data to improve comparisons between countries.

Wasting, overweight and stunting

European data from the Global Database on Child Growth and Malnutrition and from population surveys are shown in Table 2.

A prevalence of wasting greater than 5% has been documented only in Tajikistan and Uzbekistan, where it is 10–12%. Otherwise there is generally a low prevalence of wasting throughout the Region, ranging from zero and 0.8% in France and Italy in the 1970s to around 2–3% in other countries in the 1990s. Even in vulnerable groups such as refugees in Armenia and Azerbaijan, and populations under siege in Bosnia and Herzegovina *(10)*, the data indicate that protein–energy malnutrition was not a widespread public health problem.

Overweight in older children has been observed in several countries of the Region, particularly in the west. In a recent study of British schoolchildren aged 7–8 years, for example, the prevalence of overweight and obesity significantly exceeded the expected frequency *(13)*. In contrast, only a slight excess prevalence has been observed in countries in the east of the Region, such as Armenia and the Federal Republic of Yugoslavia. The Russian Federation is the exception, where 20% of young children are overweight – the highest prevalence in the Region *(11)*. Comparing obesity data for the 0–5-year-old age group is not very useful, however: while a high weight-for-age index in infancy may not be a cause for concern, since it is unlikely to continue into adulthood, obesity in the 4–5-year-old age group and older may well do so *(14,15)*.

The main nutrition-related problem in the Region is growth retardation, indicated by a low height-for-age index. The prevalence of stunting is especially high in CAR, where it affects between 7% and 43% of children under 5 years of age (Table 2). Stunting is usually most pronounced in rural areas and this is an indication of its link with environmental conditions. Such high rates of stunting are similar to those observed in African countries and should be considered a major public health problem. Intermediate values of stunting (10–22% of young children) have been observed in other CIS countries (Table 2). In contrast, the other regions all have low levels or no stunting in young children when compared with the WHO/CDC reference population.

Table 2. Prevalence of wasting, overweight and stunting in children aged 0–5 years in selected countries of the WHO European Region

Country	Year of survey	Age (years)	Wasting (%)	Overweight (%)	Stunting (%)
Balkan countries					
Bosnia and Herzegovina	1993	0–5	1.3	–	–
Croatia	1995–1996	1–6	0.8	5.9	0.8
The former Yugoslav Republic of Macedonia	1999	0–5	5.3	5.6	5.2
Federal Republic of Yugoslavia	1996	0–5 (rural)	2.2	4.8	6.8
		0–5 (urban	3.5	8.0	1.7
Central Asian republics (CAR)					
Kazakhstan	1995	0–3 (rural)	3.0	3.8	21.8
		0–3 (urban)	3.7	4.9	7.5
Kyrgyzstan	1997	0–3 (rural)	3.2	–	27.7
		0–3 (urban)	4.3	–	14.8
Tajikistan	1996	0.5–5	10.9	–	42.6
Uzbekistan	1996	0–3 (rural)	12.2	–	30.7
		0–3 (urban)	10.2	–	32.6
Central and eastern Europe					
Czech Republic	1991	0–5	2.1	4.1	1.9
Hungary	1980–1988	0–5	1.6	2.0	2.9
Romania	1991	0–5	2.5	2.3	7.8
Commonwealth of Independent States (excluding CAR)					
Armenia	1998	0–5	3.8	5.8	12.2
Azerbaijan	1996	0–5	2.9	3.7	22.2
Republic of Moldova	1996	0–5	3.2	11.7	9.6
Russian Federation	1993	0–5	3.5	20.9	17.0
Southern Europe					
Italy	1975–1977	0–6	0.8	4.4	2.7
Turkey	1993	0–5 (rural)	3.0	2.7	27.1
		0–5 (urban)	2.9	2.9	16.1
Western Europe					
France	1975	0–3	0.0	3.6	5.8
United Kingdom	1973–1979	0–5	1.0	2.9	2.4

Sources: Branca et al. *(6,7)*; Macro International *(8,9)*; Robertson et al. *(10)*; World Health Organization *(11)*; WHO/UNICEF *(12)*.

Anthropometric data for the 0–3 or 0–5-year-old range should be interpreted with caution, since they are affected by the distribution of ages within the sample. Stunting is rare during infancy and the rates of stunting are therefore usually higher if a survey includes children aged up to 5 years instead of up to 3 years. Again, there is a need to standardize the method of data collection throughout the Region in order to make useful comparisons.

Micronutrient status

The prevalence of the deficiency of four micronutrients is described here: iodine, iron and vitamins A and D. These are discussed in more detail in Chapters 4–6.

Iodine

The definition of mild, moderate and severe iodine deficiency (Table 3) is based on the combined evaluation of four different indicators: goitre in school-age children, thyroid volume greater than the 97th centile, median urinary iodine in school-age children and adults, and the prevalence of levels

Table 3. Indicators of the prevalence of iodine deficiency disorders and criteria for a significant public health problem				
Indicator	Normal	Mild deficiency	Moderate deficiency	Severe deficiency
Prevalence of goitre in school-age children	< 5%	5–19.9%	20–29.9%	> 30%
Frequency of thyroid volume in school-age children > 97th centile by ultrasound	< 5%	5–19.9%	20–29.9%	> 30%
Median urinary iodine in school-age children and adults	100–200 µg/l	50–99 µg/l	20–49 µg/l	< 20 µg/l
Prevalence of neonatal thyroid stimulating hormone above 5 µU/ml whole blood	< 3%	3–19.9%	20–39.9%	> 40%

Source: WHO Regional Office for Europe (16).

of thyroid stimulating hormone in neonates above 5 µU/ml whole blood *(16)*. Iodine deficiency disorders remain common in the European Region, as shown in Table 4.

There are clear differences in the success of public health interventions to eliminate the problem. In western European countries, iodine deficiency disorders have virtually been eliminated through universal salt iodization. In contrast, moderate levels are still found in the central Asian republics, other former Soviet countries, central and eastern Europe and Turkey. Indeed, severe or critical levels are reported in both Albania and Tajikistan. Surveys of the prevalence of goitre in schoolchildren aged 6–11 years, conducted in a range of European countries (Fig. 5), show that the highest goitre rates occur in Turkey, Belarus, Azerbaijan, the central Asian republics and even Italy. Such high goitre rates should be considered a public health priority and measures should be taken to deal with the problem.

Universal salt iodization (see Chapter 5) used to be practised in the former Soviet Union. Since the dissolution of that country, however, iodization plants are no longer in production. Although salt iodization is on the public health agenda of most of the former Soviet countries, it is not always implemented. Urinary excretion of iodine can be used to evaluate the efficiency of iodization policies; in the former Yugoslav Republic of Macedonia, for example, urinary iodine excretion has increased to normal levels as a result of salt iodization. An extensive review of the situation was carried out in the WHO European Region in 1998–1999 *(17)*.

Iron

In Europe, information on the prevalence of iron deficiency in children is limited. Most studies have investigated only the prevalence of anaemia, usually by measuring haemoblobin levels, and not its etiology, even though iron deficiency is likely to be the most common cause.

Comparison is further hindered by the use of different age groups. While some studies are carried out only in children under 3 years of age (Fig. 6), other studies go up to 5 years of age (Fig. 7). The highest prevalence of anaemia has been reported from the central Asian republics, where more than half of the children under 3 years had haemoglobin < 12 g/dl blood (Fig. 6). It should be pointed out, however, that only a small proportion of cases were of severe anaemia (haemoglobin < 7 g/dl). In western Europe anaemia is less frequent in children of this age; in the United Kingdom, for example, a 12% prevalence has been observed in children aged 1–2 years and a 6% prevalence in children aged 2–4 years. The United Kingdom

Table 4. Iodine deficiency disorders in selected European countries, according to WHO classification

Region	Virtually eliminated	Marginal and mild	Generally moderate	Severe or critical
Balkan countries		The former Yugoslav Republic of Macedonia	Croatia	Albania
Baltic countries		Estonia Latvia Lithuania		
Central Asian republics (CAR)			Kazakhstan Kyrgyzstan Turkmenistan Uzbekistan	Tajikistan
Central and eastern Europe	Slovakia	Czech Republic Hungary	Bulgaria Poland Romania	
Commonwealth of Independent States (excluding CAR)		Republic of Moldova	Armenia Azerbaijan Belarus Georgia Russian Federation Ukraine	
Nordic countries	Finland Iceland Norway Sweden			
Southern Europe			Turkey	
Western Europe	Netherlands Switzerland United Kingdom			

Source: WHO Regional Office for Europe *(16)*.

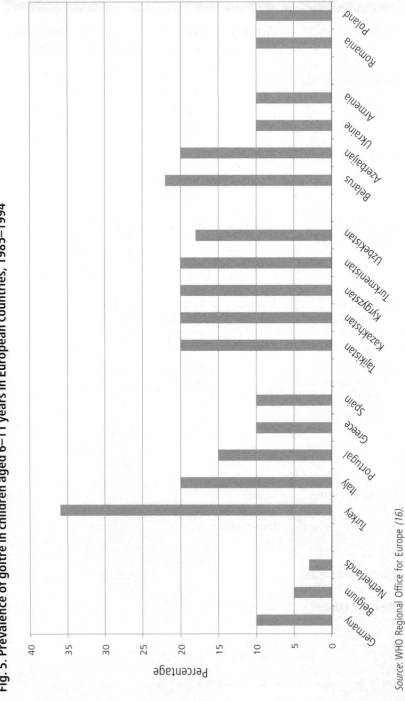

Fig. 5. Prevalence of goitre in children aged 6–11 years in European countries, 1985–1994

Source: WHO Regional Office for Europe (16).

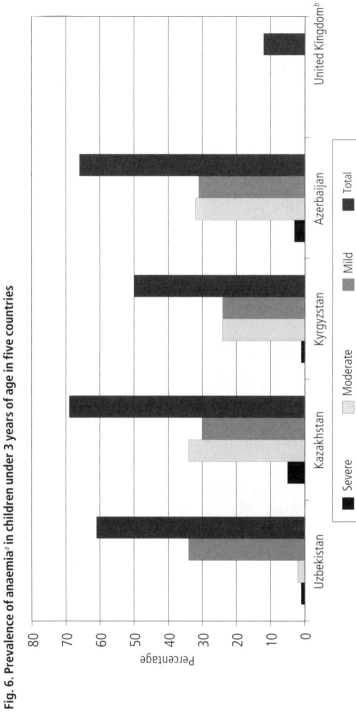

Fig. 6. Prevalence of anaemia[a] in children under 3 years of age in five countries

[a] Defined as < 12 g/dl haemoglobin.
[b] Children aged 1–2 years.
Sources: Macro International (8,9); WHO/UNICEF (12); Lawson et al. (18); Sharmanov (19).

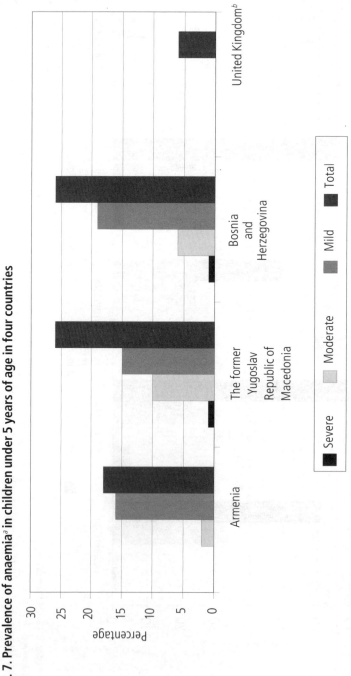

Fig. 7. Prevalence of anaemia[a] in children under 5 years of age in four countries

[a] Defined as < 12 g/dl haemoglobin.
[b] Children aged 2–4 years.

Sources: Branca et al. (6,7); Robertson et al. (10); Lawson et al. (18).

survey used a cut-off point of 11 g/dl blood; according to this, anaemia occurs in 10–30% of pre-school children living in inner cities in the United Kingdom (20). Prevalence among a nationally representative sample of Asian children living in the United Kingdom was significantly higher than this (between 20% and 45%) (18).

Factors other than iron deficiency cause anaemia. In Uzbekistan, a study of 243 children under 5 years of age showed that 72% were anaemic, but only 2% of these seemed to have non-nutritional anaemia (caused by infections and chronic diseases). In 40% of cases anaemia was associated with both low iron and low vitamin A status; 10% of cases were associated with iron deficiency alone and 20% with vitamin A deficiency alone (21).

Food intake data from the Russian Federation suggest that both women and children are at high risk of iron deficiency. Grain products rich in phytates are the major food source of iron in the Russian Federation (22). Moreover, the reported high intake of tea and low consumption of vitamin C from vegetables and fruit also compromise the bioavailability of iron present in the diet. A survey of 4077 children under 2 years of age showed a prevalence of anaemia, assessed by clinical signs, that varied from 2% (Moscow region) to 16% (Urals region). The prevalence of haemoglobin levels under 11 g/dl blood was much higher and varied from 22% (Moscow city) to 47% (Urals region). The mean haemoglobin level was significantly higher in young children in cities than in those in small towns and rural regions, at 12.2 and 11.6 g/dl, respectively (O. Netrebrenko, personal communication, 1997).

There is a shortage of studies on the cause of the high prevalence of mild to moderate anaemia in parts of eastern Europe, such as the too-early introduction of cow's milk and milk products and tea. A small study in Uzbekistan, which included measurement of ferritin and haemoglobin levels, suggested that deficiency of both iron and vitamin A was responsible. A survey carried out in Kazakhstan associated anaemia in children with stunting, morbidity and geophagia (the habit of eating soil). Geophagia was also reported from Uzbekistan (21) and is considered a symptom of iron deficiency anaemia. Clearly, further studies are needed to investigate the cause of the high prevalence of anaemia found in some parts of the European Region.

Vitamin A

Serum retinol levels under 0.35 μmol (100 μg) per litre indicate severe vitamin A deficiency; levels under 0.70 μmol (200 μg) per litre indicate low vitamin A status. A 10% prevalence of low serum retinol points to an important public health problem requiring at least public information strategies *(23)*.

There is a lack of data describing the vitamin A status of populations in the Region. Evidence suggests, however, that vitamin A deficiency is likely to be a problem in the central Asian republics. A study in the Aral Sea area of Uzbekistan showed that 40–60% of children under 5 years of age had serum retinol levels < 100 µg/l *(21)*. Another study carried out in Armenia indicated that only 0.8 % of children under 5 years of age had low levels of retinol (< 200 µg/l) *(24)*. A recent survey in the former Yugoslav Republic of Macedonia, however, showed higher levels of mild deficiency in children under 5 years: 30% had serum retinol values under 200 µg/l, but only 1% had severely low levels (< 100 µg/l) *(7)*. More information is clearly required before any policy recommendations can be made about vitamin A status in the Region.

Vitamin D deficiency and rickets

Radiographic identification of rickets has been reported in the Region, but for most countries only routine clinical data are available. One of the main causes of rickets is likely to be the traditional practice of swaddling infants, often continued until the age of 2 years, which is common in some parts of the Region. Near total covering of the skin limits its exposure to ultraviolet light and is therefore a key factor in the development of rickets. In the former Yugoslav Republic of Macedonia, 16% of children were reported to show clinical signs of rickets *(7)*. A study of 1135 Armenian children under 5 years of age *(6)* reported that 7% had an epiphyseal enlargement of the wrist, 2% had craniotabes, 25% had frontal and parietal bossing and 11% had beading of the ribs. When serum alkaline phosphatase (an indicator of vitamin D deficiency) was measured, however, only 4–6% of the children under 2 years of age had high values, indicating that rickets was no longer active in the majority. Some young children may be naturally bow-legged, thereby confounding the diagnosis of rickets; it is also unclear to what degree lack of exposure to sunlight or dietary vitamin D deficiency are responsible (see Chapter 4).

FEEDING PRACTICES AND RECOMMENDATIONS

Many countries in the WHO European Region do not have national guidelines for feeding infants and young children. Nevertheless, they do exist in several countries including Denmark, Ireland, the Netherlands, Sweden and the United Kingdom. In the former Soviet Union the need for such guidelines, which were last updated in 1982 *(25)*, was long recognized. The scientific basis underpinning optimum infant and young child feeding is still a relatively new area of research, and advances are occurring all the time. There is thus a need to ensure guidelines keep abreast of the science on which they are based.

Infant feeding recommendations appear to vary considerably between western and eastern Europe. In many countries of eastern Europe, feeding guidelines have been influenced by the recommendations of the former Soviet Union *(25)*. A review identified a number of recommendations from the former Soviet era that differ from international standards *(26)*. Poor complementary feeding practices help to explain the poor iron status and possibly the high levels of stunting among infants and young children in the European Region, and particularly in the countries of the former Soviet Union.

In relation to breastfeeding, the former Soviet literature recommended:

* late initiation of breastfeeding (up to 6–12 hours after birth), particularly in sick women and including those with anaemia;
* prelacteal feeds of 5% glucose until lactation was established;
* *exclusive* breastfeeding for the first month only (although not widely practised);
* breast-milk as the main feed for the first 4–4^1/$_2$ months;
* complete cessation of breastfeeding by 10–11 months of age; and
* breastfeeding to follow a strict timetable.

The importance of a night break between feeds was often emphasized. According to the six feeds per day regimen, a 6^1/$_2$-hour break during the night was advised; this break increased to 8 hours on the five feeds per day schedule. A review of the Soviet literature (J. Vingraité, personal communication, 1998) revealed that some authorities allowed feeds to deviate from this schedule by all of 10–15 minutes.

Non-adapted formulas in the Soviet Union included diluted fresh or fermented cow's milk with added sugar, vitamins and minerals. The introduction of cow's milk diluted with cereal water was recommended at 2–3 months (for example, 50 ml pure cow's milk or kefir, 45 ml cereal water and 5 ml 100% sugar syrup).

Former Soviet recommendations on the introduction of weaning foods included: additional fluids, primarily tea and water with sugar, for breastfed infants; the introduction of vegetable and "fruit" juices (jam with water) at

1 month of age; the introduction of unmodified cow's milk at 4 months and pure kefir at 3 months of age; the introduction of fruit at 2 months, hard boiled egg yolk at 3 months and curd at 4 months of age; the addition of sugar and salt solutions to infant foods; and the introduction of cereal porridges with added sugar, syrup, salt and butter at 4 months of age.

Of particular concern is that in cases of diagnosed anaemia (and rickets), porridge and other solids were recommended to be introduced earlier than 4 months of age.

Breastfeeding: initiation, duration and practice of exclusive breastfeeding

Owing to a lack of comprehensive and comparable data and of standardized international definitions, it is difficult to make a general statement about the prevalence of breastfeeding in the WHO European Region. The data on the percentages of breastfed infants given in Fig. 8 have been taken from different sources (27). These data should be interpreted with caution: the survey methodology varied and in some cases the way in which the surveys were carried out was not described.

With these caveats, it can be seen that the practice of breastfeeding varies dramatically between European countries. In the United Kingdom, some 25% of infants are breastfed at 3 months, compared with over 90% in Uzbekistan. Nevertheless, the prevalence of breastfeeding within a country can change dramatically over a few years. In Norway, for instance, the prevalence of breastfeeding at 3 months rose from only 25–30% in 1969 to around 80% in 1985 (28).

Unfortunately the data presented in Fig. 8 do not show the rates of "exclusive" breastfeeding. Few studies have provided a definition of "exclusive" breastfeeding, but data from those that have are presented in Fig. 9, which shows the relatively high rates of exclusive breastfeeding in Sweden both at 3 and 6 months. In contrast, the rates of exclusive breastfeeding in the central Asian republics are much lower (around 10% or less) at 3 months, except in Georgia and Kyrgyzstan where the levels are around 30%. Poland is making excellent progress: the prevalence of exclusive breastfeeding increased dramatically from almost zero in 1988 to some 40% in 1997.

In the Russian Federation in 1996 breastfeeding was initiated in about 95% of babies born in maternity hospitals (O. Netrebrenko, personal communication, 1997). The mean duration ranged from 3 to 4 months depending on when breastfeeding was initiated and on the mother's educational level.

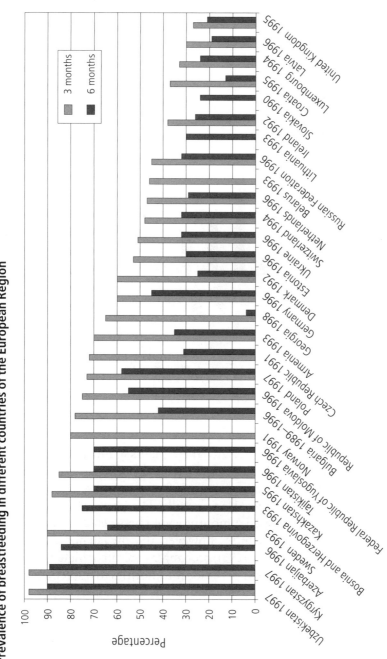

Fig. 8. Prevalence of breastfeeding in different countries of the European Region

Source: WHO Regional Office for Europe (27).

Fig. 9. Prevalence of exclusive breastfeeding in selected countries of the European Region, 1989–1998

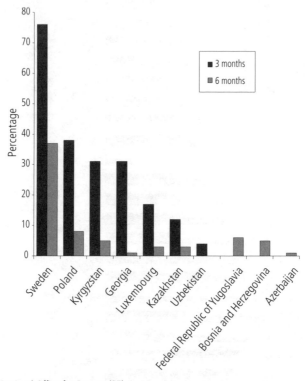

Source: WHO Regional Office for Europe *(27)*.

The most educated women breastfed their infants significantly longer than women with lower levels of education. The prevalence of partial breastfeeding was about 50% at 3 months and about 30% at 6 months. The majority of breastfed infants also received cow's milk. The prevalence of exclusive breastfeeding in infants aged 4 months varied between 22% and 28% in most regions. In St Petersburg, however, the prevalence of exclusive breastfeeding was very high (42%), probably as a result of higher education levels and of the commitment of the local authorities to implementing the international breastfeeding recommendations (see Chapter 7).

Studies in the central Asian republics indicate that, despite the high prevalence of breastfeeding, a low percentage of infants are exclusively breastfed (Fig. 9); in over 50% breastfeeding has not begun after the first 24 hours. The lack of exclusive breastfeeding, together with deteriorating socio-economic conditions, water contamination and low immunization rates, pose a threat to infant health. In Kazakhstan, despite a high level of breastfeeding with a mean duration of around 12 months, the period of exclusive breastfeeding is very short *(8)*. In the former Yugoslav Republic of Macedonia only 8% of children are exclusively breastfed at 4 months of age. Conversely, in the Nordic countries, where great efforts have been made to increase rates of exclusive breastfeeding, the percentage is very high (Fig. 8 and 9).

The rates of breastfeeding seem to be increasing throughout the Region, and the Nordic countries especially have very high rates compared with 20 years ago. Efforts should be made to maintain these high rates and greater efforts should be made in all other countries to increase rates of exclusive breastfeeding during the first few months of life (see Chapter 7). This is especially important for vulnerable groups such as ethnic minorities and low-income families living in high-risk areas with poor hygiene, sanitation and water supply.

Use of infant formulas, cow's milk and other liquids

Bottle feeding is common throughout the European Region. In Uzbekistan, 35% of children under 3 months of age examined in the 1996 Demographic and Health Survey were being fed using a bottle with a nipple, 12% to take infant formula and 23% to take evaporated milk *(9)*. In rural areas, the use of cow's milk was more common.

The early introduction of cow's milk is associated with gastrointestinal blood loss. Because the content and bioavailability of iron in cow's milk is also low, early introduction of cow's milk can lead to iron deficiency (see Chapter 6). In the Russian Federation, 12-month-old infants who received cow's milk during the first 3 months of life had significantly lower haemoglobin levels than those who received cow's milk after 7 months of age (O. Netrebrenko, personal communication, 1997). Similarly, in the United Kingdom, Asian infants are more likely than white infants to receive cow's milk and are also more likely to have iron deficiency anaemia *(29)*. Furthermore, Asian infants tend to have a higher intake of cow's milk than white children *(30)*. A study in Italy showed that, between 1983 and 1992, a reduction in the proportion of infants fed cow's milk together with an increase in breastfeeding has been paralleled by a reduction in both anaemia and iron deficiency in infants and young children *(31)*.

Table 5 shows the early introduction of cow's milk and other fluids to the infant's diet in some countries. In Lithuania, cow's milk is diluted with water or mixed with cereal water from rice, oat or buckwheat (J. Vingraité, personal communication, 1998). In Azerbaijan, wheat flour is used in combination with diluted cow's milk and egg.

Country	Average age of introduction		
	< 4 weeks	< 3 months	< 5 months

Table 5. Age of introduction of non-breast-milk fluids into the infant's diet

Baltic countries

Lithuania ... Cow's milk, goat's milk, kefir (< 5 months)

Central Asian republics (CAR)

Country	< 4 weeks	< 3 months
Kazakhstan	Water, tea with sugar	Cow's milk, tea
Kyrgyzstan	Water, tea with sugar	Cows milk, tea
Uzbekistan	Water, fruit juice	Cow's milk, tea

Commonwealth of Independent States (excluding CAR)

Country	< 4 weeks	< 3 months	< 5 months
Armenia		Water, tea	Fruit juice, cow's milk
Azerbaijan	Water, tea	Cow's milk	
Russian Federation		Fruit juice	

Western Europe

Country	< 3 months	< 5 months
United Kingdom	Herbal drink, Water	Cow's milk

Sources: Branca et al. (6); Macro International (8,9); WHO/UNICEF (12); Mills & Tyler (30).

In the Russian Federation, the types of non-breast-milk fluid given to infants differ between the large cities and the smaller towns or rural areas. In Moscow, some 50% of infants start to receive infant formula at 2 months as a supplement to breast-milk. In addition to formulas, about 10% of infants in the cities received unadapted milks (cow's milk, kefir, goat's milk) as supplements during the first 4 months. Some 22% of infants in small towns and rural areas received cow's milk or kefir at least 3 times a day during the first 4 months as a breast-milk substitute. The time of introduction of unadapted milks depended on the mother's education and the family income: infants of low-income families receive cow's milk significantly earlier than those from wealthier families (O. Netrebrenko, personal communication, 1997).

Other fluids commonly given to infants in the first or second month of life include plain or sweetened water and tea. In Uzbekistan, 40% of children received tea within the first month after birth and by 3 months of age the proportion had increased to 72% *(21)*. Other central Asian republics show similar patterns. For example, 21%, 34% and 49% of infants in Kazakhstan, Kyrgyzstan and Uzbekistan, respectively, received tea during the first few months of life *(19)*. In Armenia, water and herbal tea are introduced during the first 2 months and tea in the third month. In most instances water is boiled and given without the addition of sugar, but sugar is added to herbal tea (67%) and to ordinary tea (95%). The introduction of tea and sugar occurs even earlier in rural areas *(6)*.

The practice of giving teas (both ordinary and herbal) to infants also appears to persist in western Europe, especially among ethnic minorities, and in central Europe. This practice is not recommended, not only because it interferes with breastfeeding but also because the polyphenols present in tea impair iron absorption.

Introduction of semi-solid and solid foods

Table 6 shows the time of introduction of complementary foods in some countries. In the Russian Federation, the proportion of infants receiving foods before 4 months of age ranges from 17% in St Petersburg to 32% in the Urals region (O. Netrebrenko, personal communication, 1997). Similarly, in Armenia, children are fed semi-solid foods (crushed fruit and vegetables, porridge and potatoes) and biscuits at 4–5 months, and at 6 months they are given eggs. Bread and pasta, minced meat, fruit and vegetables are introduced at around 8–9 months of age. Other meat preparations and fish are the last to be introduced, at around 1 year of age. Compared with the Russian Federation, there appear to be fewer differences between urban and rural areas in Armenia or between residents and refugees in the age at which various foods are introduced *(6)*.

In the United Kingdom in 1996, white mothers tended to start giving their infants solid food earlier than Asian mothers. At 8 weeks, 2% of Bangladeshi, 3% of Pakistani and 5% of Indian infants had received some solid food, compared with 18% of white infants. In all groups the majority of mothers introduced food between 8 weeks and 3 months. By the age of 3 months, between 70% and 73% of Asian mothers and 83% of white mothers had given their infants some solid food *(29)*.

In the central Asian republics, infants' diets are often monotonous, mainly consisting of a porridge poor in nutrients. The results of the 1996 Demographic and Health Survey in Uzbekistan *(9)* found that 19% of 4–7-month-old infants had received meat, poultry, fish or eggs in the 24 hours preceding the interview, while 35% had received fruit or vegetables.

Table 6. Time of introduction of complementary foods into the infant's diet

Country	Average age of introduction			
	< 3 months	3–4 months	5–6 months	> 6 months
Baltic countries				
Lithuania	Fruit, berries, vegetable juice		Curd, egg yolk, oil, butter, cereals	Meat, broth
Central Asian republics (CAR)				
Uzbekistan	Vegetables, fruit	Broth	Poultry, fish, eggs, meat, flour, potatoes	Family food
Commonwealth of Independent States (excluding CAR)				
Armenia			Fruit, porridge, vegetables, potatoes, biscuits	
Azerbaijan		Potatoes, cereals, soup, milk, porridge, biscuits		
Russian Federation		Fruit	Vegetable purée, cereals	Meat
Southern Europe				
Italy		Rice porridge, fruit, parmesan	Meat, pasta, vegetables	Eggs, fish, rice, pulses
Spain			Cereals, fruit	Bread, vegetables, yoghurt, meat, fish, eggs, pulses

Sources: Branca et al. *(6)*; Macro International *(9)*; WHO/UNICEF *(12)*; Ferrante et al. *(32)*; Savino et al. *(33)*; Van den Boom et al. *(34)*.

In the Balkan region, Albanian infants receive diets based heavily on cereals *(35)* and in the former Yugoslav Republic of Macedonia diets include large amounts of grain, beans and vegetables. The socioeconomic situation affects nutritional status by decreasing the ability to buy meat and milk products due to their high price *(36)*. Thus the introduction of fruit and vegetables, and of meat and liver may be delayed or reduced by economic and/or seasonal factors. In contrast, meat is introduced at 5–6 months in Italy and after 6 months in Spain.

REFERENCES

1. PELLETIER, D.L. The relationship between child anthropometry and mortality in developing countries: implications for policy, programs and future research. *Journal of nutrition*, **124**: 2047S–2081S (1994).
2. *Measuring change in nutritional status.* Geneva, World Health Organization, 1983.
3. *Prevention and control of iron deficiency anaemia in women and children. Report of the UNICEF/WHO Regional Consultation, Geneva, 3–5 February 1999.* Geneva, United Nations Children's Fund, 1999.
4. *Central and eastern Europe in transition: public policy and social conditions. Poverty, children and policy: responses for a brighter future.* Florence, UNICEF International Child Development Centre, 1995 (Economies in Transition Studies, Regional Monitoring Report, No. 3).
5. *Health and health care.* Yerevan, Ministry of Health of Armenia, 1997.
6. BRANCA, F. ET AL. *The health and nutritional status of children and women in Armenia.* Rome, National Institute of Nutrition, 1998.
7. BRANCA, F. ET AL. *Mulitiple indicator cluster survey in Fyrom with micronutrient component.* Rome, National Institute of Nutrition, 1999.
8. *Kazakstan Demographic and Health Survey, 1995.* Calverton, MD, Macro International Inc., 1996.
9. *Uzbekistan Demographic and Health Survey, 1996.* Calverton, MD, Macro International Inc., 1997.
10. ROBERTSON, A. ET AL. Nutrition and immunisation survey of Bosnian women and children during 1993. *International journal of epidemiology*, **24**: 1163–1170 (1993).
11. *WHO global database on child growth and malnutrition.* Geneva, World Health Organization, 1997 (document WHO/NUT/97.4).
12. *Nutrition survey of children under 5 of Azerbaijan.* Geneva, World Health Organization and United Nations Children's Fund, 1997.
13. REILLY, J.J. ET AL. Prevalence of overweight and obesity in British children: a cohort study. *British medical journal*, **319**: 1039 (1999).

14. ROLLAND-CACHERA, M.F. ET AL. Increasing prevalence of obesity among 18-year-old males in Sweden: evidence for early determinants. *Acta paediatrica*, **88**: 365–367 (1999).

15. ROLLAND-CACHERA, M.F. ET AL. Influence of adiposity development: a follow-up study of nutrition and growth from 10 months to 8 years of age. *International journal of obesity and related metabolic disorders*, **19**: 573–578 (1995).

16. DELANGE, F. ET AL., ED. *Elimination of iodine deficiency disorders (IDD) in central and eastern Europe, the Commonwealth of Independent States and the Baltic states. Proceedings of a conference held in Munich, Germany, 3–6 September 1997.* Copenhagen, WHO Regional Office for Europe, 1998 (document WHO/EURO/NUT/98.1).

17. *Comparative analysis of progress on the elimination of iodine deficiency disorders.* Copenhagen, WHO Regional Office for Europe, 2000 (document EUR/ICP/LVNG 01 01 01).

18. LAWSON, M.S. ET AL. Iron status of Asian children aged 2 years living in England. *Archives of disease in childhood*, **78**: 420–426 (1998).

19. SHARMANOV, A. Anaemia in central Asia: demographic and health service experience. *Food and nutrition bulletin*, **19**: 307–317 (1998).

20. GREGORY, J.R. ET AL. *National diet and nutrition survey children aged 1.5–4.5 years. Vol 1. Report of the diet and nutrition survey.* London, H.M. Stationery Office, 1995.

21. MORSE, C. *The prevalence and causes of anemia in Muynak District, Karakalpakistan, the Republic of Uzbekistan.* Brandon, MS, Crosslink International, 1994.

22. KOHLMEIER, L. Deficient dietary iron intakes among women and children in Russia: evidence from the Russian Longitudinal Monitoring Survey. *American journal of public health*, **88**: 576–580 (1998).

23. *Indicators for assessing vitamin A deficiency and their application in monitoring and evaluating intervention programmes.* Geneva, World Health Organization, 1996 (document WHO/NUT/96.10).

24. UNITED NATIONS CHILDREN'S FUND. *Infant feeding in Armenia. Report on a comparative study and national survey.* Yerevan, American University of Armenia, 1997.

25. *Infant feeding. Methodical recommendations.* Moscow, Ministry of Health of the USSR, 1982.

26. *Complementary feeding and the control of iron deficiency anaemia in the Newly Independent States: presentation by WHO at a WHO/UNICEF consultation, Geneva, Switzerland, 4 February 1999.* Copenhagen, WHO Regional Office for Europe, 2000.

27. *Comparative analysis of implementation of the Innocenti Declaration in WHO European Member States. Monitoring Innocenti targets on the protection,*

promotion and support of breastfeeding. Copenhagen, WHO Regional Office for Europe, 1999 (document EUR/ICP/LVNG 01 01 02).

28. HEIBERG ENDERSEN, E. & HELSING, E. Changes in breastfeeding practices in Norwegian maternity wards: national surveys 1973, 1982 and 1991. *Acta paediatrica*, **84**: 719–724 (1995).

29. THOMAS, M. & AVERY, V. *Infant feeding in Asian families.* London, Stationery Office, 1997.

30. MILLS, A. & TYLER, H. *Food and nutrient intakes of British infants aged 6–12 months.* London, H.M. Stationery Office, 1992.

31. SALVIOLI, G.P. Iron nutrition and iron stores changes in Italian infants in the last decade. *Annali del'Istituto Superiore di Sanità*, **31**: 445–459 (1995).

32. FERRANTE, E. ET AL. Retrospective study on weaning practice in Rome and interland. Results and comment. *Minerva pediatrica*, **46**: 275–283 (1994).

33. SAVINO, F. ET AL. Weaning practice in Torinese area: epidemiological study on practice and age of introduction of complementary food. *Minerva pediatrica*, **46**: 285–293 (1994).

34. VAN DEN BOOM, S.A.M. ET AL. Weaning practices in children up to 19 months of age in Madrid. *Acta paediatrica*, **84**: 853–858 (1995).

35. BARDHOSHI, A. ET AL. Country report – Albania. Development of local food based dietary guidelines and nutrition education. *In: Workshop on Development of Local Food Based Guidelines and Nutrition Education, Nitra, Slovakia, 22–25 September 1997.* Rome, Food and Agriculture Organization of the United Nations, 1997.

36. PETRUSEVSKA-TOZI, L. ET AL. Country report – Macedonia. Development of local food based dietary guidelines and nutrition education. *In: Workshop on Development of Local Food Based Guidelines and Nutrition Education, Nitra, Slovakia, 22–25 September 1997.* Rome, Food and Agriculture Organization of the United Nations, 1997.

CHAPTER 2

Recommended nutrient intakes

Each country should use recommended nutrient intakes for infants and young children, based on international scientific evidence, as the foundation of its nutrition and feeding guidelines.

INTRODUCTION

This and the next four chapters include discussion and comparison of the recommended nutrient intakes (RNIs) from the European Union, the United Kingdom, the United States and WHO. These values provide a standard against which the adequacy of the diets of young children, as measured by food intake surveys, can be assessed *(1)*.

The purpose of RNIs is to provide guidance for policy-makers on how much of each nutrient is needed to ensure that a population is healthy (Box 1). The aim is to prevent deficiency (for example, iodine to prevent goitre); to optimize health (for example, recommendations for anti-oxidants in vegetables and fruit); and to provide safe limits above which a nutrient (for example, excess protein or energy) could be harmful.

Box 1. Applications and limitations of recommended nutrient intakes

1. RNIs provide a benchmark for the development of dietary guidelines and the planning of public health nutrition strategies.

2. RNIs can be useful for food labelling (for example, a food might be described as containing x% of the recommended intake of vitamin C for a given age group).

3. RNIs can be used to assess and interpret dietary surveys and food intake information relating to normal healthy populations.

4. RNIs can be used to assess the adequacy of the dietary intake of vulnerable groups.

Source: adapted from Weaver *(2)*.

Additional factors such as bioavailability (of iron, for example) must be taken into consideration when setting national RNIs.

RECOMMENDATIONS ARE DERIVED FROM REQUIREMENTS

A requirement is defined as the lowest continuing level of intake of a nutrient that will maintain a defined level of nutrition in an individual *(3)*. The actual nutrient requirement will vary from individual to individual, whereas a nutrient recommendation must cover the requirements of almost all those in a given population. RNIs are useful for assessing the diet of groups within a population, not of individual children, and recommendations must take account of the large biological variation within a population. The metabolic needs of healthy individuals, such as the needs for growth, are taken into account whereas the increased nutrient demands of illness are not.

In the United Kingdom, a committee convened by the Department of Health *(4)* decided to use the term "dietary reference values" rather than RNIs. The committee chose to set, where possible, three values for each nutrient, reflecting a range of nutrient requirements (low, medium and high) (Fig. 10) rather than just one value. These three values, known collectively as dietary reference values, include the mean value (the "estimated average requirement"), the mean value plus two standard deviations (the "reference nutrient intake") and the mean value minus two standard deviations (the "lower reference nutrient intake"). An example of this approach is shown in Table 7, where the three values are presented for zinc.

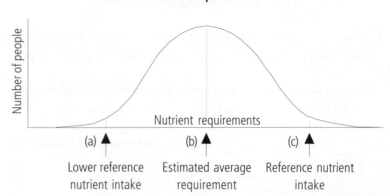

Fig. 10. Relationship between various reference values for nutritional requirements

Table 7. Dietary reference values (mg/day) for zinc in the United Kingdom			
Age of child	Lower reference nutrient intake	Estimated average requirement	Reference nutrient intake
0–3 months	2.6	3.3	4.0
4–6 months	2.6	3.3	4.0
7–9 months	3.0	3.8	5.0
10–12 months	3.0	3.8	5.0
1–3 years	3.0	3.8	5.0
4–6 years	4.0	5.0	6.6

Source: Department of Health, United Kingdom (4).

Underlying the concept for defining recommendations is the assumption that the requirements of most nutrients are distributed normally in a population (Fig. 10). The level that is sufficient to meet the requirements of practically all the population is set at the upper end of the distribution at approximately two standard deviations above the mean. This recommendation, the reference nutrient intake, should cover the nutrient requirements of approximately 95% of the population, whereas the mean value will meet those of around half the population. Because excess intake of energy leads to obesity, the mean value is the recommended value for energy; the higher value would undoubtedly lead to excess energy intake in a large percentage of the population and increase the risk of obesity-related diseases. The value at the lower end of the distribution curve is estimated by calculating the mean minus two standard deviations. If the habitual mean intake of a population were at the level of the lower reference nutrient intake, more than half the population would be deficient in that particular nutrient and thus their complete nutrient requirements would not be satisfied.

Most estimates are derived from a limited number of balance studies or intake surveys, and care is therefore required in interpreting RNIs. For example, RNIs for infants are often based on measures of the breast-milk intake of exclusively breastfed infants. Between the ages of 6 and 12 months, and sometimes up to 24 months, nutrient recommendations are derived by extrapolating from the data for this younger age group, using a formula that allows for growth and increasing body size. The nutrient recommendations for children aged over 24 months are in most cases extrapolated from adult values, on the assumption that children have a similar maintenance requirement for a given nutrient per kilogram of body weight. To most of these recommendations is added an additional increment as a safety margin in order to protect against any risk of deficiency.

NOMENCLATURE OF RECOMMENDED NUTRIENT INTAKES

Several countries have established their own RNI systems, and different nomenclatures are used (Table 8). The European Union uses population reference intakes (PRI) and the former Soviet Union used the term "physiological norm". The RNIs used in this publication correspond to the reference nutrient intake shown in Fig. 10. It should be noted that the abbreviation "RNI" used here, unless otherwise stated, refers to recommended and not reference nutrient intake.

The criteria presented in Box 2 reflect the fact that the RNI is usually set around the mean value representative of a group, plus two standard deviations. However, the trend is to consider the optimal intake of each nutrient as opposed to setting levels designed only to prevent deficiency. This includes considering the problem of excess nutrient intakes, such as of energy, protein, vitamin A, vitamin D and iron, which are potentially harmful if regularly consumed in excessive amounts.

Table 8. Definitions of nutrient recommendations		
Source	**Name**	**Definition**
European Union	Population reference intake (PRI)	The intake that will meet the needs of nearly all healthy people in a group (5).
United Kingdom	Reference nutrient intake (RNI)	An amount of the nutrient that is enough, or more than enough, for about 97% of people in a group (2).
United States	Recommended dietary allowances (RDA)	The levels of intake of essential nutrients that, on the basis of scientific knowledge, are judged ... to be adequate to meet the known nutrient needs of practically all healthy persons (6).
	Adequate intake (AI)	

Source: Weaver *(2).*

Box 2. Criteria used for setting nutrient recommendations

- The amount taken by a group of people without deficiency developing.
- The amount needed to cure deficiency.
- The amount needed to maintain enzyme saturation.
- The amount needed to maintain blood or tissue concentration.
- The amount associated with an appropriate biological marker of adequacy.

RNIs are based on limited scientific information and it must be borne in mind that values have changed over the years. For example, the United Kingdom's 1979 estimates of energy requirements during infancy *(7)* were lowered by the 1991 Committee *(4)*. This was because, based on new evidence *(8,9)*, it was no longer considered necessary to overestimate energy requirements to allow for the possible underestimation of breast-milk intake. Similarly, it appears that in the former Soviet Union the level of protein recommended was much higher than that recommended in western Europe.

Because there is so much inter-individual variation, it is difficult to predict the true nutrient requirements of an individual without substantial and lengthy nutritional and clinical assessment. The actual requirement of the individual is likely to be less than the RNI. Thus, comparing the actual intake of an individual against reference data only provides information on the likelihood that his or her nutrient requirements are within the range of intakes recommended for the population.

No attempt is made in the following chapters to define new RNIs. Rather, those of the European Union, the United Kingdom, the United States and WHO (where these exist) are presented so that the range of values can be compared. Where no national values exist, or if countries wish to update their current RNIs, the values presented here provide an overview and a basis on which to develop national RNIs and dietary guidelines.

REFERENCES

1. AGGET, P.J. ET AL. Recommended dietary allowances (RDAs), recommended dietary intakes (RDIs), recommended nutrient intakes (RNIs), and population reference intakes (PRIs) are not "recommended intakes". *Journal of pediatric gastroenterology and nutrition*, **25**: 236–241 (1997).

2. WEAVER, L.T. Nutrition. *In*: Campbell, A.G.M. et al., ed. *Forfar & Arneil's textbook of paediatrics*, 5ᵗʰ ed. Edinburgh, Churchill Livingstone, 1992, pp. 1179–1180.

3. US INSTITUTE OF MEDICINE. *Dietary reference intakes for thiamin, riboflavin, niacin, vitamin B_6, folate, vitamin B_{12}, pantothenic acid, biotin, and choline.* Washington, DC, National Academy Press, 1998.

4. DEPARTMENT OF HEALTH, UNITED KINGDOM. *Dietary reference values for food energy and nutrients for the United Kingdom. Report of the Panel on Dietary Reference Values of the Committee on Medical Aspects of Food Policy.* London, H.M. Stationery Office, 1991 (Report on Health and Social Subjects, No. 41).

5. EUROPEAN COMMISSION. *Report of the Scientific Committee on Food (thirty-first series). Nutrient and energy intakes for the European Community.* Luxembourg, Office for Official Publications of the European Communities, 1993.

6. US NATIONAL RESEARCH COUNCIL. *Recommended dietary allowances*, 10th ed. Washington, DC, National Academy Press, 1989.

7. DEPARTMENT OF HEALTH, UNITED KINGDOM. *Recommended daily amounts of food energy and nutrients for groups of people in the United Kingdom.* London, H.M. Stationery Office, 1979 (Report on Health and Social Subjects, No. 15).

8. PRENTICE, A.M. ET AL. Are current guidelines for young children a prescription for overfeeding? *Lancet*, 2: 1066–1069 (1988).

9. LUCAS, A. ET AL. How much energy does a breast-fed infant consume and expend? *British medical journal*, 295: 75–77 (1987).

Energy and macronutrients

Provision of adequate dietary energy is vital during the period of rapid growth in infancy and early childhood. Attention must be paid to feeding practices that maximize the intake of energy-dense foods without compromising micronutrient density.

An adequate protein intake with a balanced amino acid pattern is important for the growth and development of the infant and young child. If the child receives a varied diet, however, protein quantity and quality are seldom a problem. It is prudent to avoid a high-protein diet because this can have adverse effects.

During complementary feeding and at least until 2 years of age, a child's diet should not be too low (because this may diminish energy intake) or too high in fat (because this may reduce micronutrient density). A fat intake providing around 30–40% of total energy is thought to be prudent.

Consumption of added sugars should be limited to about 10% of total energy, because a high intake may compromise micronutrient status.

ENERGY

Function

Energy is required for tissue maintenance and growth, to generate heat (thermogenesis) and for physical activity. Weight gain is a sensitive indicator of the adequacy of energy intake in young children. The energy requirement is the amount of dietary energy needed to balance the energy expended and that deposited in new tissue (growth). Energy expenditure can be subdivided into basal metabolism, which represents 50–60% of total energy expenditure (TEE) in most healthy children, energy expended on physical activity (30–40% of TEE in most healthy children) and thermogenesis (approximately 5–8% of TEE). The energy required for growth declines rapidly from around 35% of TEE at birth to 5% at 1 year (Fig. 11). Basal metabolic rate can be considered to represent a "maintenance" requirement, since it is the energy cost of biosynthesis, metabolism and the physical work of respiratory and cardiac function. The energy expended on physical activity varies widely, while that expended on thermogenesis is primarily the cost of digesting, absorbing and resynthesizing nutrients.

Fig. 11. Comparison of energy requirements during infancy and adulthood

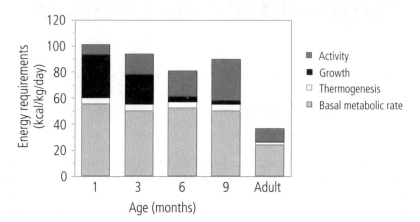

Growth demands some energy expended on biosynthesis, in addition to the energy content of newly synthesized tissue.

Sources
Dietary energy is consumed in the form of fat, carbohydrate and protein. Fat accounts for approximately 50% of the energy in breast-milk and is the main source of energy for infants less than 6 months old. With the introduction of complementary food, fat is gradually overtaken by carbohydrate as the chief energy source, and together they meet the energy needs of the growing child. Dietary protein can also be oxidized to provide energy, but its primary role is in the growth and maintenance of new tissues. Per unit of body weight, the intakes of energy, fat and carbohydrates of the normal infant during the early months of life are far greater than the corresponding intakes of normal adults (Fig. 12). This is because the maximum rate of growth occurs in infancy, when the baby doubles its body weight in the first 6 months and triples it by 1 year.

Per unit body weight, the intake of energy by an exclusively breastfed infant is 2.3 times that of an adult. Compared with an adult, and calculated per gram of macronutrient, an infant's intake of protein is almost the same, the intake of fat almost four times and the intake of carbohydrate almost double.

Requirements
Current WHO recommendations for energy intake for the first 12 months of life *(1)* were based on the observed average energy intakes of healthy children in affluent countries, plus a 5% increment for an assumed underestimation of breast-milk intake.

Fig. 12. Daily energy intake and energy sources in an exclusively breastfed infant aged 3–4 months (6.3 kg) and an adult male (70 kg) with moderate physical activity eating a recommended diet[a]

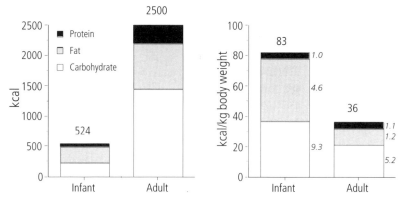

[a] The values in italic to the right of the columns in the right-hand figure indicate the intake of macronutrients in g/kg body weight.

Butte *(2)* reviewed relevant literature published since 1985 to develop updated estimates of energy requirements of both exclusively breastfed and formula-fed infants. These were based on energy intake, TEE measured using the doubly labelled water technique, and the energy required for growth (tissue deposition). These updated energy requirements are considerably lower than the earlier recommendations *(1)* (Table 9) and suggest that current recommendations may overestimate infant energy requirements by 15–30%.

Both sets of figures in Table 9 show a fall in energy intake per kg body weight between 3 and 6 months, which is maintained until 9 months and then rises again towards 1 year. This reduction reflects the period when the very high growth rate characteristic of the first 3 months of life has declined but is not yet balanced by increased physical activity.

Table 10 provides an overview of the estimated energy requirements recommended by the United Kingdom, the United States, the European Union and WHO for infants and children of different ages. These values are derived from estimated energy requirements per kg body weight multiplied by an average body weight for the age range. There is considerable similarity between them, and therefore these international comparisons could form the basis for recommendations in countries seeking to develop their own standards or physiological norms for energy.

Table 9. Estimated energy requirements in kJ (kcal)/kg body weight

WHO (1)		Butte (2)[a]	
Age (months)	Estimated energy requirement	Age (months)	Estimated energy requirement
0.5	519 (124)	0–1	364 (87)
1–2	485 (116)	1–2	376 (90)
2–3	456 (109)	2–3	380 (91)
3–4	431 (103)	3–4	345 (83)
4–5	414 (99)	4–5	339 (81)
5–6	404 (96.5)	5–6	334 (80)
6–7	397 (95)		
7–8	395 (94.5)	6–9	347 (83)
8–9	397 (95)		
9–10	414 (99)		
10–11	418 (100)	9–12	372 (89)
11–12	437 (104.5)		

[a] Based on energy required for total energy expenditure plus growth of breastfed infants.

Table 10. Recommended nutrient intakes for energy in MJ (kcal)/day

Age	United Kingdom	United States	European Union	WHO
Boys				
0–3 months	2.3 (545)	2.7 (650)	2.2 (525)	2.3 (545)
4–6 months	2.9 (690)	2.7 (650)	3.0 (715)	2.9 (690)
7–9 months	3.4 (825)	3.5 (850)	3.5 (835)	3.4 (825)
10–12 months	3.9 (920)	3.5 (850)	3.9 (930)	3.9 (920)
1–3 years	5.2 (1230)	5.4 (1300)	5.1 (1215)	5.2 (1230)
4–6 years	7.2 (1715)	7.5 (1800)	7.1 (1690)	7.2 (1715)
Girls				
0–3 months	2.2 (515)	2.7 (650)	2.1 (500)	2.2 (515)
4–6 months	2.7 (645)	2.7 (650)	2.8 (670)	2.7 (645)
7–9 months	3.2 (765)	3.5 (850)	3.3 (790)	3.2 (765)
10–12 months	3.6 (865)	3.5 (850)	3.7 (880)	3.6 (865)
1–3 years	4.9 (1165)	5.4 (1300)	4.8 (1140)	4.9 (1165)
4–6 years	6.5 (1545)	7.5 (1800)	6.7 (1595)	6.5 (1545)

Source: Garrow et al. (3).

For girls and boys aged less than 2 years, reference nutrient intakes are assumed to be identical when expressed per unit body weight. Owing to their greater average weight, therefore, boys have higher estimated average requirements for energy.

Physical activity

Energy requirements change with physical activity and under stressful environmental conditions, such as extremes of temperature and during illness, but precise estimates of the range of these variations are not available for infants and young children. Physical activity plays a key role in the psychological and social development of young children and it is therefore essential that children receive adequate energy to support optimal physical activity. There is some evidence that when energy intake is insufficient, activity may be reduced to maintain growth (4).

Energy required from complementary foods

The energy needed from complementary foods depends on the energy obtained from breast-milk and the energy requirements of the individual infant. It is therefore difficult to estimate the average energy required from complementary foods alone. In the WHO/UNICEF report on complementary feeding in developing countries (5), however, an attempt was made to estimate this.

The energy needed from complementary foods can be calculated by subtracting the energy consumed as breast-milk from the recommended energy intake. Values used for the recommended energy intake are those proposed by Butte (2) (Table 9) for infants aged up to 12 months, and by Torun et al. (6) for young children aged 12 months and over. Estimates of mean breast-milk intake were derived from a comprehensive review of the published literature from both developing and industrialized countries, and from both exclusively and partially breastfed infants. Energy requirements were assumed to be the same for all these groups of infants.

Because the mean intake of breast-milk was slightly lower in developing than in industrialized countries, the energy needed from complementary foods in the 3–8-month age group in developing countries is slightly higher (Table 11). The original theoretical analyses (5) include a range of high to low intakes of breast-milk (mean ± 2 standard deviations). The range is wide and, for example in industrialized countries, values range from zero to 1.7 MJ/day (408 kcal/day) in the 6–8-month age group.

The data given in Table 11 suggest that infants from industrialized countries, with an average breast-milk intake, do not require any complementary

Table 11. Age-specific estimates of energy in MJ (kcal)/day required from complementary foods in industrialized and developing countries, assuming an average breast-milk intake				
Age group (months)	**Industrialized countries**		**Developing countries**	
	Breast-milk	**Complementary foods**	**Breast-milk**	**Complementary foods**
0–2	2.1 (490)	0.0 (0)	1.8 (437)	0.0 (0)
3–5	2.3 (548)	0.0 (2)	2.0 (474)	0.3 (76)
6–8	2.0 (486)	0.8 (196)	1.7 (413)	1.1 (269)
9–11	1.6 (375)	1.9 (455)	1.6 (379)	1.9 (451)
12–23	1.3 (313)	3.3 (779)	1.5 (346)	3.1 (746)

Source: World Health Organization (5).

food to meet their energy requirements until the age of 6–8 months, when they need 0.8 MJ (196 kcal)/day from complementary food. As mentioned, however, the range of needs is wide and it is vital to interpret these estimates cautiously. The actual energy requirements of each infant will depend on his or her body weight and other factors, including rate of growth.

In contrast, it appears that a 3–5-month-old infant from a developing country does need a small amount of energy from complementary food (0.3 MJ (76 kcal)/day). This figure is the difference between the energy needs of an infant with a median body weight according to the WHO reference and energy from a breast-milk intake based on available data from developing countries, where infants often have a low body weight; the figure may therefore be inflated. Furthermore, studies suggest that the introduction of complementary foods before 6 months is likely to displace breast-milk (7,8) and its early introduction is thus not effective in increasing the total energy intake.

Thus, after about 6 months of age, breast-milk alone does not meet a child's energy needs, and appropriate complementary foods are necessary to supply the additional energy required. The evidence for when to introduce complementary foods is reviewed in more detail in Chapter 8.

Low intake
If energy intake is less than the energy requirement of the individual, physical activity and/or rate of growth will be reduced. If the deficit continues,

protein–energy malnutrition will develop. Low energy intake may also result in the metabolism of protein for energy and consequently protein deficiency (see page 54).

High intake

When energy intake exceeds requirements, fat deposition and weight gain increase. However, fat deposition during infancy is part of normal growth. The rate of fat deposition, measured as subcutaneous fat or body fat, is very fast up to the age of 4 months, and slows thereafter until the age of about 6 years. Fat mass as a percentage of body mass increases until about 6 months of age and gradually declines thereafter. Total fat, on the other hand, is on average higher in a 6-year-old than a 1-year-old, although it will be lower per unit of body weight.

Studies from the early 1970s suggested that fatness during infancy could result in a lifelong risk of obesity. More recent epidemiological studies, however, show no strong correlation between fatness during infancy and obesity in later life *(9,10)*. It is now generally agreed that fatness during infancy is not a risk factor for obesity later in life. Nevertheless, the degree to which fatness during early childhood (second and third years of life) is associated with obesity in later life is not known. Given the escalating prevalence of obesity in the Region, it is prudent to limit fat and sugar intake and thereby energy intake from the age of 2–3 years. Furthermore, all children should be encouraged to be physically active.

ENERGY DENSITY

Infants and young children have an energy intake per kg body weight some 2–3 times that of adults (Fig. 11 and 12). Because they have to ingest large amounts of energy, a key determinant of energy intake is the energy density of complementary foods. Too low an energy density may result in an energy deficit and consequently poor growth. The amount of energy an infant can eat is determined by a number of factors (Fig. 13). Energy density is increased by raising the content of fat and sugar, while a higher water content will decrease energy density. Energy intake is increased through complementary food with a high energy density, more frequent meals and an increased intake of breast-milk. Conversely, energy intake will be reduced if complementary foods are very viscous, which is typically the result of a high starch content.

Energy intake is also influenced by functional gastric capacity, which determines the volume of food an infant can ingest during one meal. The

Fig. 13. Factors affecting the energy density of complementary foods and energy intake by the infant and young child.
The direction of influence is indicated as positive (+) or negative (–).

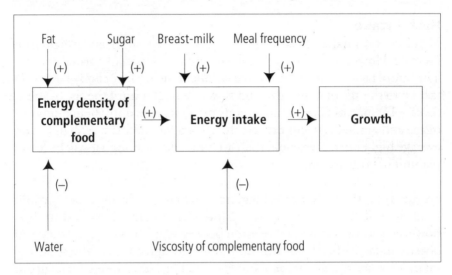

functional gastric capacity is determined not only by the volume of the stomach but also by its rate of emptying. If the energy density of a meal is low, the infant will require a large volume of food to satisfy energy requirements, and this may exceed the infant's gastric capacity. Functional gastric capacity has been estimated to be about 30 g/kg body weight (5). This is equal to values of approximately 250, 285 and 345 g/meal for infants of average body weight at 6–8, 9–11 and 12–23 months, respectively. These estimates of gastric capacity were used to calculate the minimum energy density of complementary food (5). Table 12 shows the energy densities needed to satisfy energy requirements assuming an average breast-milk intake (see Table 11) or no breast-milk intake and different meal frequencies. These figures depend on a number of assumptions about gastric capacity, and the number and composition of meals, and should therefore be regarded as rough estimates.

Based on these data, the WHO/UNICEF report (5) concluded that breastfed infants older than 8 months should receive at least three meals of complementary foods per day and that, if the energy density of the diet is less than 4.2 kJ (1 kcal)/g, more than three meals are needed. Furthermore, the report recommended that for those infants receiving little or no breast-milk (or suitable alternative formula), at least four meals per day, or very energy-dense food, are required. Studies of the dietary intake of infants and young

Table 12. Minimum energy density in kJ (kcal)/g of complementary foods by number of meals per day, breast-milk intake and age group

Age range (months)	Average breast-milk intake			No breast-milk		
	2 meals	3 meals	4 meals	2 meals	3 meals	4 meals
6–8	3.8 (0.9)	2.5 (0.6)	1.6 (0.4)	7.1 (1.7)	4.6 (1.1)	3.8 (0.9)
9–11	5.0 (1.2)	3.4 (0.8)	2.5 (0.6)	7.5 (1.8)	5.0 (1.2)	3.8 (0.9)
12–23	6.3 (1.5)	4.2 (1.0)	2.9 (0.7)	8.4 (2.0)	5.4 (1.3)	4.2 (1.0)

Source: World Health Organization (5).

children from industrialized countries show that the energy density of the total diet (breast-milk combined with complementary foods) slowly increases from that of breast-milk (2.8 kJ (0.67 kcal)/g) (11). The average energy density of complementary foods is higher than that of breast-milk; if it falls below that of breast-milk, studies suggest that the total energy intake will be too low. It is therefore prudent to assume that the average energy density of complementary foods should be at least 2.8 kJ (0.67 kcal)/g and ideally closer to 4.2 kJ (1 kcal)/g.

Energy density varies considerably among different complementary foods. Foods with a high energy density include meat and fatty fish. Most complementary foods, however, are based on a staple that is high in complex carbohydrates, and therefore bulky and viscous, often with a low energy and nutrient density. Porridges, for example, typically have a very low energy density (< 2.1 kJ (< 0.5 kcal)/g) if they are prepared without milk or fat. To reduce their viscosity and thereby make them easier for infants and young children to consume, water is often added to complementary foods, particularly to porridges. This further reduces their energy and nutrient density, and is therefore not recommended.

There are several ways in which the energy density of a complementary food can be increased. Adding fat or sugar increases the energy density without increasing the viscosity of the food (Fig. 13). Fat is most efficient because it is very energy-dense (38 kJ (9 kcal)/g) while sugar, like other carbohydrates and protein, contains only 17 kJ (4 kcal)/g. Both fat and sugar, however, contain no protein and almost no micronutrients and thus the nutrient density of the meal will be reduced. The amount of fat that can be added to a diet without reducing the intake of micronutrients to a level below the recommended intake depends on the total micronutrient content of the diet.

National recommendations from industrialized countries advise a dietary fat content of about 35–45% total energy intake for the age group 6–12 months, decreasing to about 30–40% from 12 months to 2–3 years of age *(12)*. In contrast, it is recommended *(5)* that in developing countries fat intake should be lower, at approximately 30% of total energy intake (25% in the complementary diet). This last recommendation is based on a concern that if a high quantity of fat is added to a monotonous cereal-based diet with a borderline micronutrient content, then this low micronutrient content would be further diluted. In the present report, a fat intake providing around 30–40% of total energy is thought to be prudent for the first 2 years of life.

PROTEIN
Function
Proteins are the major functional and structural components of all the body's cells. They are diverse in structure and function: enzymes, blood transport molecules, the intracellular matrix, fingernails and hair are all composed of proteins, as are most hormones and components of membranes. Amino acids, the building-blocks of proteins, also act as precursors for the synthesis of many coenzymes, hormones, nucleic acids and other molecules essential for life. Thus, to maintain cellular integrity and function and to ensure health and growth, an adequate supply of dietary protein is vital. Proteins may also be a source of energy during times of energy deprivation, although fat and carbohydrate are utilized preferentially by the body.

Protein intake is particularly important in infancy and childhood, when rapid growth requires amino acids from which to build new tissue (particularly the organs and muscle). All amino acids provide nitrogen for synthesis of human proteins, but some essential (indispensable) amino acids cannot be synthesized by the body and must therefore be supplied in the diet. If deprived of these essential amino acids, the body will catabolize its own proteins to produce them. Adequate intakes of essential amino acids can be achieved so long as the diet contains a variety of protein sources (see below). In adults, the essential amino acids are isoleucine, leucine, lysine, methionine, phenylalanine, threonine, tryptophan, valine and histidine. Arginine is an essential amino acid for children. Cysteine, taurine and tyrosine appear to be essential amino acids for the preterm infant, but evidence is inconclusive as to their essentiality for term infants.

The body can synthesize other amino acids from simple precursors, and these are termed the nonessential amino acids. They are alanine, aspartic acid, cysteine, glutamic acid, glycine, proline, serine and tyrosine. There are only very small reserves of protein in the body (approximately 3% of the total body content), and therefore pathological conditions such as starvation, injury or infection can cause substantial rates of protein loss from the body protein mass. Protein is catabolized mainly by the breakdown of muscle cells to provide the necessary amino acids, or energy if energy intake is low, to maintain protein synthesis. Thus if dietary sources of nitrogen are limited, all amino acids become "essential". If breast-milk (or other milk) intake is significant, however, the need for essential amino acids from complementary foods is very small, and nitrogen can be provided from plant proteins as long as there is sufficient energy.

Sources

Good sources of high-quality protein include animal sources, such as liver, meat, fish, cheese, milk and eggs, and some vegetable sources, primarily soya products, green beans and pulses. Wheat products are also good sources of vegetable protein, but most vegetables and fruit contain little protein.

Proteins are classified nutritionally according to the quantity and proportion of essential amino acids that they contain. The biological value of a protein refers to its ability, when it is the sole dietary source of protein, to support protein synthesis and therefore body maintenance and growth. On this scale, breast-milk proteins and egg have the highest value, 1.0. All animal proteins (with the exception of gelatin) are complete, that is they contain all the essential amino acids and are of high biological value. Most vegetable proteins, except soya, are incomplete because they offer an unbalanced assortment of amino acids that cannot alone satisfy the body's needs. An essential amino acid supplied in less than the amount needed to support protein synthesis is known as a limiting amino acid; in cereal diets, for example, lysine tends to be limiting. This so-called "limiting" can be overcome by mixing different vegetable protein sources together, as explained in Chapter 8.

Because proteins are digested to amino acids or small peptides before they are absorbed, it is the mixture of amino acids derived from the ingested foods that is important. Protein complementation is the process by which a protein of low biological value, lacking amino acid X but containing Y, is eaten with another low-value protein, rich in X but not Y, the two together giving a good mix of amino acids equal to a protein of high biological value. Thus, if cereals are consumed with milk proteins, which have a high lysine content, there is significant complementation and the limiting factor is overcome.

Coeliac disease

Coeliac disease is the result of a sensitivity in a small number of children to dietary gluten, a protein that causes injury to the mucosa of the small intestine, leading to malabsorption and other clinical problems including iron deficiency and wasting. Gluten is a mixture of proteins found in cereals, and it is the gliadin fraction of gluten that is toxic to the intestinal epithelium, precipitating gluten enteropathy or coeliac disease. The gliadin content of wheat is considerably higher than that of other cereals. Gliadin itself is a mixture of proteins, and research is under way to identify the different epitopes and mechanisms by which they cause mucosal damage.

Coeliac disease sometimes manifests itself during the complementary feeding period, after the infant first encounters foods containing gluten. It may take some time to develop clinically, and if genetically predisposed individuals are breastfed and are not introduced to gluten-containing foods until after 6 months of age, the onset of the disorder will probably be delayed or possibly prevented. This delay may be important, because nutrition and growth will not be compromised during the particularly vulnerable stage of rapid growth. New data from Sweden suggest that not only breastfeeding, but also the age at which gluten is introduced into the diet and the amount of gluten consumed in early life, affect the risk of developing coeliac disease *(13)*. Coeliac disease is treated by lifelong exclusion of gluten from the diet. Most countries recommend that infants should not receive gluten-containing foods before 6 months of age. Thus, it seems prudent to recommend that gluten-containing cereals should not be introduced before the age of about 6 months.

Requirements

The 1985 recommendations on protein requirements for infants less than 6 months of age *(1)* were based on intake data from breastfed infants. It was concluded that the protein requirements of infants up to 6 months of age will be fully satisfied as long as energy needs are met and the food offered contains protein in a quantity and quality equivalent to that in human milk. Not all of the protein in human milk is "nutritional", as some functional proteins such as secretory IgA can be found in the stools. Nevertheless, although the protein requirement per unit of body weight is greater in infants than in any other age group, the nitrogen from breast-milk is highly bioavailable and well absorbed and is matched by a high energy intake per unit of body weight. This concept can be illustrated by the energy and protein requirements of a 3-month-old infant. Breast-milk is perfectly adapted to infant needs and is relatively low in protein compared with cow's milk. At 3 months of age, protein intake represents approximately 5–6% of total energy intake compared with about 10–15% in adults. With an average daily breast-milk intake of around 800 ml, the protein requirements (estimated at 1.4 g/kg body weight/day) will be satisfied.

Table 13 shows that the protein requirements for infants aged 2–5 months, as estimated in 1985 *(1)*, were 7–19% greater than the intakes of exclusively breastfed infants estimated by Dewey et al. *(14)*. The most probable explanation for this difference is that protein requirements were overestimated in 1985.

The 1985 estimates of mean protein requirements used a modified factorial approach, based on estimates of maintenance nitrogen needs and those for growth, which in children under 2 years is a significant percentage. Lack of data and dependence on certain assumptions limit these estimates, and there is a need for more evidence on which to base reliable recommendations of the safe level of protein intake for children, particularly during the critical period of rapid growth in the first 12 months. In the absence of evidence from direct experimentation, protein requirements are based on an estimate of the protein intake that would meet the mean requirement; a safe level is then set at two standard deviations above this in order to meet the needs of the vast majority of infants. Estimates for safe protein requirements in infants aged 0–12 months are shown in Table 13. National and international recommendations are based on these estimated requirements (Table 14).

The former Soviet "physiological norms" for protein were significantly higher (over three times in some cases) than levels recommended by international expert committees. As a result, studies investigating the adequacy

Table 13. Estimated protein "requirements" in g/kg body weight/day for infants aged 0–12 months		
Age (months)	**FAO/WHO/UNU *(1)***	**Dewey et al. *(14)***
0–1	–	2.69
1–2	2.25	2.04
2–3	1.82	1.53
3–4	1.47	1.37
4–5	1.34	1.25
5–6	1.30	1.19
6–9	1.25	1.09
9–12	1.15	1.02

Table 14. Recommended nutrient intakes for protein in g/day[a]				
Age	United Kingdom	United States	European Union	WHO
0–3 months	12.5	13	–	12.5
4–6 months	12.7	13	14.0	12.7
7–9 months	13.7	14	14.5	13.7
10–12 months	14.9	14	14.5	14.9
1–3 years	14.5	16	14.7	14.5
4–6 years	19.7	24	19.0	19.7

[a] Recommended protein intake per day is calculated by multiplying recommended protein intakes per kg body weight with the mean body weight for infants in each age group.

Source: Garrow et al. (3).

of protein intakes in the former Soviet countries may erroneously claim to find widespread protein deficiency. Indeed, there is very little evidence to support claims that widespread protein deficiency exists in any of the former Soviet countries, including the central Asian republics.

Low intake
Protein deficiency is almost always accompanied by inadequate energy intake, and the two together give rise to protein–energy malnutrition, one of the commonest forms of malnutrition worldwide. In children, acute protein–energy malnutrition (caused by recent severe food deprivation) is characterized by a low weight-for-height index (wasting), while the chronic condition (caused by long-term food deprivation) is characterized by a low height-for-age index (stunting). Severe protein–energy malnutrition results in the clinical syndromes of marasmus, kwashiorkor or marasmic kwashiorkor. All three conditions are compounded by a range of nutritional disorders, including micronutrient deficiencies (15).

In infants and young children in industrialized countries, severe malnutrition is usually secondary to gastrointestinal disorders or chronic systemic disease such as tuberculosis, cystic fibrosis or cancer. Nevertheless, primary malnutrition unrelated to illness may be caused by insufficient food availability, lack of care or poverty. Specific causes include: formula feeds that are overdiluted; home-made formulas of inappropriate composition; prolonged partial breastfeeding without adequate addition of complementary foods; excessive juice intake; the offering of inadequate food because of perceived food "allergens"; and the inappropriate provision of a milk-free diet that is low in protein.

High intake

Family foods tend to contain a high proportion of protein (approximately 10–15% of total energy intake) and if the diet is low in fat the percentage of total energy intake contributed by protein can be between 15% and 20%. Such protein intakes are 3–4 times greater than the protein requirements of infants and young children.

Diets high in protein offer no benefits and can theoretically have a number of adverse effects. High circulating blood levels of amino acids may exceed the capacity of the hepatic and renal systems to metabolize and excrete the excess nitrogen. This may lead to acidosis, diarrhoea and elevated levels of blood ammonia and urea. The high potential renal solute load associated with diets rich in protein reduces the margin of safety related to the maintenance of water balance. Consequently, during periods of illness with associated dehydration, the reduced capacity to excrete waste products increases the risk of hypernatraemia. High prevalence of hypernatraemic dehydration has virtually disappeared in some countries, probably as a result of the higher rates of breastfeeding and the use of modified cow's milk formula with lower protein and salt content *(16)*.

In addition to the risk that high protein intakes can compromise fluid balance, excess protein intake has also been linked to obesity in later life. In a longitudinal study of children, for example, those with a high protein intake at the age of 2 years had a significantly higher risk of being obese at 8 years *(17)*. However, this association is not proven to be causal.

FAT

Function

Dietary fats provide the infant and young child with energy, essential fatty acids and the fat-soluble vitamins A, D, E and K. Fats also heighten the palatability of food, thereby promoting greater energy intake. Furthermore, several fatty acids, especially the long-chain polyunsaturated fatty acids, have specific and essential physiological functions.

The different types of fat (structural and storage) in the body have diverse functions, and the quality as well as the quantity of fat intake is important. The structural fats are mainly constituents of cell membranes and neural tissue and thereby contribute to the architecture of cells, while the storage fats act as a long-term reserve of metabolic fuel for the body. The largest store of fatty acids that supply long-term energy needs is adipose tissue, which is principally composed of triglycerides. Similarly breast-milk fat, which is the main energy source for young infants, is 98% triglycerides. Triglycerides are the richest source of energy and have an energy density of 38 kJ (9 kcal)/g, which is more than twice that of carbohydrate or protein.

Sources

Dietary fat includes all of the lipids found in both plant and animal foods (Table 15). In nutritional terms, fats are often divided into "visible" fats, such as cooking oils, butter and the fat on meats, and "invisible fats", which are those incorporated into foods during preparation and cooking (for example in cakes and biscuits), or present in processed meats and sausages and emulsions such as mayonnaise. The majority of both visible and invisible fats are triglycerides, but fats may also be present in plant membranes and animal tissues, and these are chiefly phospholipids, glycolipids and cholesterol. Fats from animal produce (for example, cow's milk and meat) tend to contain saturated fatty acids, while those from plants and fish tend to contain monounsaturated or polyunsaturated fatty acids (Table 15). In adults, saturated fats are associated with an increase in cardiovascular diseases, but there are no data to suggest that saturated fat intake during the first years of life contributes to this problem. In contrast, unsaturated fat consumption is associated with a lower prevalence of cardiovascular disease in adults.

There are two essential fatty acids, linoleic and α-linolenic acids, that the human body cannot synthesize. These are precursors of phospholipids, prostaglandins and the long-chain polyunsaturated fatty acids, including arachadonic and docosahexaenoic acids. Young infants have limited ability

Table 15. Dietary fats and their sources	
Dietary factor	**Typical sources**
Saturated fatty acids	Butter, lard, cow's milk fat, cheese, meat and sausages
Monounsaturated fatty acids	Olive, canola and rapeseed oils
Polyunsaturated fatty acids	
Linoleic acid	Corn, sunflower, soya and safflower oils
α-linolenic acid	Fish oils, soya oil and fats in vegetables and nuts
Trans fatty acids	Hydrogenated fat in margarines, biscuits and cakes
Dietary cholesterol	Eggs, meat, butter and whole milk

to synthesize arachadonic and docosahexaenoic acids but both are present in human milk. Most commercial infant formulas do not contain docosahexaenoic acid, and the membrane phospholipids in the brains of infants whose intake of this fatty acid is deficient have replaced it with other fatty acids. Docosahexaenoic acid is a major constituent of the developing brain, and its replacement with other fatty acids is likely to change the functional characteristics of neural cells *(18)*.

Requirements
About 50% of the energy available in human milk is derived from fat. Many foods adapted for infants have a substantially lower proportion of their energy derived from fat *(12)*, and thus the proportion of total dietary energy provided as fat gradually decreases as a wider variety of foods are introduced. When defining an optimal level of dietary fat during the period of complementary feeding, it is vital to ensure that there is enough fat to meet the requirements for essential fatty acids, and that energy density is within a desirable range.

It has therefore been recommended *(12)* that, during the complementary feeding period (between about 6 and 24 months), a child's diet should derive 30%–40% of energy from fat. This translates into a total energy intake of approximately 3% from linoleic acid and approximately 0.3% from linolenic acid. However, the optimal intake of long-chain polyunsaturated fatty acids for this age group remains controversial.

Fat can make a considerable contribution to the energy density of the mixed diet and, because it does not normally increase the viscosity of food, it can be used to increase energy density without resulting in an overly thick preparation. However, the fat content should not be so great as to displace protein or micronutrients or to induce gastrointestinal intolerance.

Low intake
Infants and young children have particularly high energy requirements for their body weight. To safeguard growth during this period, therefore, restricted diets and especially low-fat diets (those with a low energy density) should not be recommended for this age group. In support of this, there is some epidemiological evidence to suggest that poor growth during early life might increase the risk of cardiovascular disease later in life *(19)*.

High intake
The main rationale for restricting fat intake during childhood is to prevent obesity and cardiovascular disease later in life. Evidence for a beneficial

effect of a lower fat intake during infancy and early childhood on later cardiovascular disease is indirect, however, and is based primarily on extrapolation from studies of adults and children with hypercholesterolaemia. The atherosclerotic vascular lesions found before puberty are reversible. Although high blood lipid levels during early childhood tend to continue to be relatively high, there is no proof that lowering fat intake during early life reduces the risk of developing cardiovascular disease later in life (20). Furthermore, epidemiological studies have shown that infant obesity is a poor predictor of obesity later in childhood and in adulthood (17,21).

CARBOHYDRATES

Function

Carbohydrates provide a significant proportion of the energy in the human diet. Ultimately, all carbohydrates in food are converted to and absorbed as monosaccharides, primarily glucose. Glucose is an essential fuel for all body tissues and particularly the brain, which is unable to metabolize fat for energy. Under normal conditions, a rise in blood glucose above a certain level leads to its removal from the circulation and storage as glycogen in the liver or muscle, or conversion into and storage as fat.

Glycoproteins are polypeptides containing short chains of carbohydrates, and are present in many tissues. Glycoproteins are involved in a range of functions, and include the mucins that provide a protective lining for epithelia, particularly that of the gut.

The colon is inhabited by a large and complex bacterial microflora, which is capable of fermenting most of the carbohydrate that has not been digested and absorbed in the small intestine. This unabsorbed carbohydrate (starches and non-starch polysaccharides) is fermented to lactic acid and short-chain fatty acids, including acetic, propionic and butyric acids, and to gases that include hydrogen, carbon dioxide and methane.

Short-chain fatty acids represent a source of energy for the colonic mucosa and other body tissues, and it is estimated that in adults fermentation generates at least 2 kcal per gram of unabsorbed carbohydrate. Furthermore, short-chain fatty acids have important health benefits. Butyric acid is the principal fuel for colonocytes and may help to prevent colonic disease, while propionic and acetic acids may have positive effects on liver metabolism and on general energy balance, respectively. Moreover, short-chain fatty acids are rapidly absorbed, promoting water absorption and thereby reducing the risk of osmotic diarrhoea.

Sources

Dietary carbohydrates include sugars (with up to 3 monosaccharide units), oligosaccharides (with up to 10 monosaccharide units) and complex carbohydrates (starches and fibres with 10 or more monosaccharide units). Sugars are soluble carbohydrates, comprising mainly monosaccharides such as glucose, fructose and galactose and disaccharides such as sucrose, lactose and maltose. Starches are composed of polysaccharide chains and have physical states that are subject to modification by cooking. The polysaccharides (excluding starch) form a complex group of polymers mainly derived from plant cell walls, and are the principal components of "dietary fibre".

Sugars

Sugars can be classified into two groups: those that are naturally integrated into the cellular structure of food (the most important being whole fruits and vegetables containing mainly fructose, glucose and sucrose) and those that are not located within the cellular structure of the food, and either exist free in food or are added to it. Free or added sugars can be subdivided further into the milk sugars (mainly lactose, representing around 37% of the energy in human milk) that naturally occur in milk and milk products, and all other sugars (added sugars). These include refined sugar (sucrose) from sugar cane and beet (used in recipes, at the table or in soft drinks) and honey (a mixture of fructose and glucose).

Sugars provide energy but they make no other contribution to nutrient needs. Infants enjoy the taste of sweet foods, and parents may be tempted to use them as a comfort or reward. It is thus important that the infant diet should offer a variety of tastes and textures, and that infants should not come to expect that their food and drink will always be sweet (see Chapter 8, pages 180–181). Unsweetened cereals, yoghurts and kefir should be preferred to those containing a large quantity of sugar. There is no advantage in terms of dental health of replacing sucrose with other sweet foods such as honey or fructose.

Starch

Complementary feeding should, as a priority, ensure adequate energy. Although starch is well tolerated and relatively efficiently digested and absorbed, a starch-rich diet tends to be bulky. Cooked cereal products and vegetables provide suitable sources of starch in the infant's diet. Rice starch is well digested and absorbed and is particularly suitable during early complementary feeding because it is gluten-free. Data on starch intakes by infants and young children are scarce, but it is generally recommended that an increasing starch intake with age should be encouraged provided that the total energy intake remains adequate.

Dietary fibre

Dietary fibre can be defined as the non-starch polysaccharides (cellulose, hemicellulose A and B, gums, mucilages and pectins) and lignin. A common characteristic of all dietary fibres is that they are not fully digested in the small intestine and they enter the colon where they are available for fermentation by the colonic microflora.

The principal positive effect of fibre in children is probably that of regulating bowel movement. Some forms of dietary fibre are better than others for increasing stool weight and frequency, softening faeces, increasing faecal bulk and reducing gastrointestinal transit time. Constipation can be prevented and treated with dietary fibre. The effects appear to vary according to the type of fibre consumed: insoluble, coarsely ground fibre has a more marked effect in retaining water, and thereby increasing stool frequency, than finely ground soluble fibre. The products of the bacterial fermentation of dietary fibre may also directly affect bowel habit.

Fibre may prevent or be used to treat obesity. High-fibre foods have a lower energy density, satisfy hunger, "flatten" the post-prandial glycaemic response and slow the rates of food ingestion, gastric emptying and digestion. However, there are very few useful studies of these effects in children. In older children, no adverse effects have been reported from the consumption of fibre-containing foods, and there is no information available from developing countries where higher fibre intakes frequently coexist with low energy intake.

Foods used for complementary feeding should not in general contain as much fibre as the adult diet, because fibre can displace the energy-rich foods that children under 2 years of age need for growth. Infants and young children who receive diets with inappropriately high amounts of low-energy-density foods may not have an adequate energy intake, which can result in failure to thrive.

Fruit and vegetables are good for older infants and young children. They are rich in fibre and are also good sources of micronutrients and other beneficial substances. Many foods rich in fibre, however, such as whole-grain cereal products and legumes, also contain phytates, which impair the absorption from the diet of zinc and iron.

Research is needed on foods that promote a beneficial colonic flora. From the second year of life, progressive introduction of natural foods in the form of vegetables, (whole) cereals, legumes and fruit will accustom the infant to a balanced and correct dietary habit within a mixed diet. Indeed, these recommendations would help to control the overconsumption of protein found in the 12–24-month period in most countries *(21)*.

Requirements

Provided energy is adequate, starch intake should gradually increase with a concomitant decrease in fat intake. Added sugars represent "empty calories", being a source of energy only and not associated with any micronutrients. Thus, a diet with a high proportion of energy from added sugars has a reduced capacity to ensure micronutrient needs and may cause diarrhoea (this is particularly true of fructose-rich fruit drinks). Several countries recommend that the intake of added sugars should not exceed 10% of total energy intake, equal to approximately five level teaspoons (25 g) of sugar per day for a 12-month-old infant. This figure is arbitrary and studies do not recommend it specifically. However, given that there are no benefits of a high intake of added sugars, it seems prudent to keep this figure as a recommendation. If added sugars are consumed in excess of about 30% of total energy intake, undesirable elevations in plasma concentrations of glucose, insulin and lipids may occur *(22)*. Such intakes should be avoided, and children with intakes of this magnitude should replace the excess with starch and nutrient-rich foods, especially fruit and vegetables. Reducing added sugar intake should also lower the risk of dental caries in preschool children.

Low intake

A low energy intake depletes glycogen and adipose stores, and thereafter increases the risk of hypoglycaemia. Although glucose can be synthesized by the liver from amino acids and propionic acid, a minimum amount of dietary carbohydrate is essential to inhibit ketosis (the accumulation of ketoacids formed in the liver from fatty acids) and to allow complete oxidation of fat.

High intake

Diets high in fibre are energy-sparse and bulky, and diets over-rich in fibre are therefore not recommended for infants and young children. Children over 2 years of age, for whom an energy-dense diet is of less concern, should be encouraged to eat foods rich in complex carbohydrates, since these play a vital role in normal bowel function. There is very little evidence that excess carbohydrate intake is a cause of obesity in infancy.

REFERENCES

1. *Energy and protein requirements. Report of a joint FAO/WHO/UNU expert consultation.* Geneva, World Health Organization, 1985 (WHO Technical Report Series, No. 724).

2. BUTTE, N.F. Energy requirements of infants. *European journal of clinical nutrition,* **50** (Suppl. 1): S24–S36 (1996).

3. GARROW, J.S. ET AL., ED. *Human nutrition and dietetics,* 10th ed. London, Churchill Livingstone, 1999.

4. WATERLOW, J.C. Energy-sparing mechanisms. Reductions in body mass, BMR and activity: their relative importance and priority in undernourished infants and children. *In:* Schürch, B. & Scrimshaw, N.S. *Activity, energy expenditure and energy requirements of infants and children.* Lausanne, International Dietary Energy Consultative Group, 1990.

5. *Complementary feeding of young children in developing countries: a review of current scientific knowledge.* Geneva, World Health Organization, 1998 (document WHO/NUT/98.1).

6. TORUN, B. ET AL. Energy requirements and dietary energy recommendations for children and adolescents 1 to 18 years old. *European journal of clinical nutrition,* **50** (Suppl. 1): S37–S80 (1996).

7. SIMONDON, K.B. ET AL. Effect of early, short-term supplementation on weight and linear growth of 4–7-month-old infants in developing countries: a four-country randomized trial. *American journal of clinical nutrition,* **64**: 537–545 (1996).

8. COHEN, R.J. ET AL. Effects of age of introduction of complementary foods on infant breast milk intake, total energy intake, and growth: a randomised intervention study in Honduras. *Lancet,* **344**: 288–293 (1994).

9. ROLLAND-CACHERA, M.F. ET AL. Tracking the development of adiposity from one month of age to adulthood. *Annals of human biology,* **14**: 219–229 (1987).

10. ROBERTS, S.B. Early diet and obesity. *In:* Heird, W.C., ed. *Nutritional needs of the six to twelve month old infant.* New York, Raven Press, 1991.

11. MICHAELSEN, K.F. & JØRGENSEN, M.H. Dietary fat content and energy density during infancy and childhood: the effect on energy intake and growth. *European journal of clinical nutrition,* **49**: 467–483 (1995).

12. *Fats and oils in human nutrition. Report of a joint expert consultation.* Rome, Food and Agriculture Organization of the United Nations, 1994 (FAO Food and Nutrition Paper, No. 57).

13. IVARSSON, A. ET AL. Epidemic of coeliac disease in Swedish children. *Acta paediatrica,* **89**: 165–171 (2000).

14. DEWEY, K.G. ET AL. Protein requirements of infants and children. *European journal of clinical nutrition,* **50** (Suppl. 1): S119–S150 (1996).

15. *Management of severe malnutrition: a manual for physicians and other senior health workers*. Geneva, World Health Organization, 1999.
16. ARNEIL, G.C. & CHIN, K.C. Lower solute milks and reduction of hypernatraemia in young Glasgow infants. *Lancet*, **2**: 840 (1979).
17. ROLLAND-CACHERA, M.F. ET AL. Influence of adiposity development: a follow-up study of nutrition and growth from 10 months to 8 years of age. *International journal of obesity and related metabolic disorders*, **19**: 573–578 (1995).
18. COCKBURN, F. Neonatal brain and dietary lipids. *Archives of disease in childhood, fetal and neonatal edition*, **70**(1): F1–F2 (1994).
19. BARKER, D.J.P., ED. *Fetal and infant origins of adult disease*. London, British Medical Journal, 1992.
20. ESPGAN COMMITTEE ON NUTRITION. Committee report: comment on childhood diet and prevention of coronary heart disease. *Journal of pediatric gastroenterology and nutrition*, **19**: 261–269 (1994).
21. ROLLAND-CACHERA, M.F. ET AL. Increasing prevalence of obesity among 18-year-old males in Sweden: evidence for early determinants. *Acta paediatrica*, **88**: 365–367 (1999).
22. DEPARTMENT OF HEALTH, UNITED KINGDOM. *Dietary sugars and human disease*. London, H.M. Stationery Office, 1989 (Report on Health and Social Subjects, No.37).

CHAPTER 4

Vitamins

In countries where there is a high prevalence of childhood infectious disease, it is important to determine whether vitamin A deficiency is a public health problem.

In countries where rickets is a public health problem, all infants should receive a vitamin D supplement as well as adequate exposure to sunlight.

In this chapter, the vitamins that are most relevant to the health of infants and young children in the European Region are discussed. The RNIs of those vitamins that are not discussed here (vitamins E and K, and the B vitamins thiamin, riboflavin, niacin, vitamin B_6, biotin and pantothenic acid) are given in the Appendix to this chapter. Table 16 shows the main sources and functions of vitamins.

VITAMIN A
Function
Vitamin A is required for healthy vision, for the integrity of epithelial surfaces, and for the development and differentiation of tissues. It is also essential for embryonic development and many other physiological processes, including spermatogenesis, normal immune response, taste, hearing and growth. In addition, several carotenoids including β-carotene, which can be converted into vitamin A, appear to act as important antioxidants in tissues. Together with vitamin C and vitamin E they deactivate or scavenge free radicals (highly reactive molecules) and activated oxygen, and may therefore protect against cellular damage. β-carotene is also involved in maintaining an effective immune response.

Sources
Vitamin A is obtained as preformed retinol from animal products or is converted from the carotenoids, in particular β-carotene, present in plant food. Levels of preformed vitamin A are highest in liver, dairy products, eggs and fish. Dark green leafy vegetables and yellow vegetables (such as carrots) and fruit are rich sources of carotenoids. The consumption of foods rich in vitamin A should be encouraged once complementary feeding has started.

Requirements and RNIs
In order to express vitamin A requirements in units that allow for the differing potency of retinol and the carotenoids, the unit "retinol equivalents"

Table 16. The main sources and functions of vitamins

Vitamin	Important sources	Functions
Vitamin A (retinol)	Liver, dairy products, fish oils, orange and green vegetables, fortified margarines	Eyesight Healthy skin and mucous lining of body organs
Vitamin D (cholecalciferol)	Fish oils, salmon, herring, liver, skin exposure to UV light	Bone formation
Vitamin E (tocopherol)	Vegetable oils, whole grain cereals, nuts, seeds, green leafy vegetables	Antioxidant properties, protecting cells from oxidative damage
Vitamin K	Colonic bacteria	Blood clotting
Vitamin C (ascorbic acid)	Citrus fruits, peppers, tomatoes, cabbage	Formation of supporting tissues of cells for wound healing Absorption of non-haem iron
Vitamin B_1 (thiamin)	Whole grain cereals and breads, legumes, nuts, meat	Carbohydrate utilization
Vitamin B_2 (riboflavin)	Green leafy vegetables, meat, eggs, milk	Nervous system function Protein metabolism Growth
Vitamin B_3 (niacin or nicotinic acid)	Whole grain cereals, nuts, legumes, meat, poultry, fish	Energy metabolism
Vitamin B_{12} (cyanocobalamin)	Meat, eggs, fish, poultry, milk, roots/nodules of legumes (otherwise not generally present in plants)	Red blood cell formation Nervous system function

Table 16 (contd)		
Vitamin	**Important sources**	**Functions**
Folic acid	Yeast, liver, kidneys, green leafy vegetables, orange juice	To aid maturation of red blood cells
Vitamin B$_6$ (pyridoxine)	Liver, kidneys, meat, whole grain cereals, egg yolk	Protein metabolism Formation and growth of red blood cells
Biotin	Liver, egg yolk, soya flour, cereals, yeast	Cofactor for gluconeogenesis and fat metabolism
Pantothenic acid	Animal products, whole grains, legumes	Essential for numerous reactions involved in lipid and carbohydrate metabolism

(RE) has replaced International Units (IU). 1 µg retinol is equivalent to 1 RE, and it takes 6 µg β-carotene to form 1 RE (1 RE = 3.33 IU vitamin A).

Infants are born with vitamin A stores in the liver and these, together with intakes of vitamin A from breast-milk, will satisfy requirements until about 6 months of age. The amount of vitamin A secreted in breast-milk depends on maternal intake and stores. If the vitamin A status of the mother is sufficient, breast-milk is also an important source of vitamin A after the age of 6 months. However, mothers deficient in vitamin A may not provide enough of it in their milk to build up infant liver stores or to protect the infant from deficiency beyond 6 months of age (1). For children in populations with a high prevalence of vitamin A deficiency, complementary foods are an important source of vitamin A after 6 months of age.

International recommendations for vitamin A intake (Table 17) are remarkably consistent, and suggest that intakes of around 350–400 RE per day should meet the needs of all healthy infants and young children.

Low intake
Infants and young children are vulnerable to the adverse effects of both deficiency and excess of vitamin A. Xerophthalmia, the result of severe

Table 17. Recommended nutrient intakes for vitamin A in RE/day				
Age	United Kingdom	United States	European Union	WHO safe level [a]
0–3 months	350	375	–	350
4–6 months	350	375	–	350
7–9 months	350	375	–	350
10–12 months	350	375	–	350
1–3 years	400	400	400	400
4–6 years	400	400	400	400

[a] Safe level = upper end of normative storage requirement.

Source: Garrow et al. (2).

prolonged vitamin A deficiency, is a major preventable cause of child-hood blindness in many countries of the developing world. In the WHO European Region, overt clinical vitamin A deficiency does not seem to be a problem, although data on the prevalence of vitamin A deficiency in the Region are limited. In Uzbekistan, 40–60% and in Armenia around 1% of children under 5 years of age had serum retinol values below 0.35 µmol (100 µg)/l, indicating severe deficiency (3,4). In the former Yugoslav Republic of Macedonia, 30% of children under 5 years had mild vitamin A deficiency (serum retinol values below 0.70 µmol (200 µg)/l) (5).

Evidence suggests that mild vitamin A deficiency without clinical signs is associated with an increased susceptibility to infection, and intervention studies suggest that vitamin A supplementation of deficient populations can reduce mortality (6) and morbidity from infectious diseases (7). Furthermore, vitamin A deficiency is a contributing factor to anaemia. The above-mentioned study carried out in Uzbekistan (3) reported that 40% of anaemic children under 5 years had low iron and low vitamin A status, and 20% had low vitamin A status only. There is an interaction between vitamin A and iron. In populations with deficiencies of both nutrients, supplementation with iron will have a positive effect on vitamin A status and vice versa (8). Recent studies suggest that as well as correcting iron deficiency, improvement in vitamin A status will have a positive effect on iron status.

In populations with a high prevalence of vitamin A deficiency, high priority should be given to reducing it because of its association with morbidity, anaemia and mortality. Maternal status should be improved through dietary intervention or daily supplements. Breastfeeding should be encouraged because breast-milk is a good source of vitamin A, and foods rich in vitamin A should be given during the complementary feeding period. Where it is not feasible to make such interventions within a reasonable time, supplementation in areas with moderate or severe vitamin A deficiency should be considered. A high dose should be given at intervals of 3–6 months or, if daily vitamin D supplements are already available, a combined vitamin A and D supplement should be given.

High intake

Toxic effects, including bone and liver damage, may arise following a single very large dose of retinol or from the ingestion of excessive doses of vitamin A supplements over a long period. Daily intakes of retinol should not exceed 900 RE in infants and 1800 RE in children between 1 and 3 years of age *(9)*.

B VITAMINS

This section on the B vitamins will focus only on folic acid and vitamin B_{12} (Tables 18 and 19). Deficiency of both of these vitamins can cause megaloblastic anaemia. It is not known what proportion of anaemia can be attributed to folic acid and/or vitamin B_{12} deficiency in the Region. The relationship is difficult to elucidate as there are many nutritional and non-nutritional causes of anaemia. Thus, further research and surveys are needed to describe the epidemiology of folic acid and vitamin B_{12} deficiency.

Table 18. Recommended nutrient intakes for folic acid in µg/day				
Age	United Kingdom	United States	European Union	WHO safe level[a]
0–3 months	50	25	50	16
4–6 months	50	25	50	24
7–9 months	50	35	50	32
10–12 months	50	35	50	32
1–3 years	70	50	100	50
4–6 years	100	75	130	50

[a] Based on normative storage requirement with 15% coefficient of variation.

Source: Garrow et al. *(2)*.

Table 19. Recommended nutrient intakes for vitamin B_{12} in µg/day				
Age	United Kingdom	United States	European Union	WHO safe level
0–3 months	0.3	0.3	–	0.1
4–6 months	0.3	0.3	–	0.1
7–9 months	0.4	0.5	0.5	0.1
10–12 months	0.4	0.5	0.5	0.1
1–3 years	0.5	0.7	0.7	0.5
4–6 years	0.8	1.0	0.9	0.8

Source: Garrow et al. *(2)*.

The main symptoms of folic acid deficiency are megaloblastic anaemia, poor appetite, weight loss and failure to thrive. Both human milk and cow's milk are good sources (40–60 µg/l). Folic acid is heat-labile, however, and megaloblastic anaemia responsive to folic acid supplementation has been described in infants given heat-treated home-made cow's milk formula or unfortified commercial infant formula *(10)*.

Children consuming a macrobiotic diet are at risk of vitamin B_{12} deficiency, and infants breastfed by strict vegan mothers are at risk of impaired neurological development, anaemia and even encephalopathy.

Sources
Folic acid occurs in leafy vegetables and also in liver, beans, beetroot, wholemeal bread, eggs and some fish.

The richest source of vitamin B_{12} is liver. Other sources include shellfish, fish, meat, eggs, milk, cheeses and yoghurt.

VITAMIN C
Function
Vitamin C is essential for the prevention of scurvy and for the promotion of wound healing. Furthermore, it is important for the optimal functioning of the immune system and for the synthesis of collagen, and it has antioxidant properties. Vitamin C is particularly valuable in assisting the absorption of non-haem iron from vegetables and other non-haem sources

(see Chapters 6 and 8). This is probably achieved by chelation with iron to form a soluble compound that readily releases iron to the intestinal mucosa. The enhancing effect of vitamin C on the absorption of iron, and probably of zinc, from a meal depends on the presence of adequate amounts of vitamin C. For example, consuming food containing 25 mg ascorbic acid will approximately double the amount of iron absorbed from cereals (11). To be effective, foods and drinks rich in vitamn C should be consumed at the same time as foods containing non-haem iron, to allow the necessary conversion of ferrous iron to ferric iron.

Sources
Vegetables and fruit, especially spinach, tomatoes, potatoes, broccoli, berries, oranges and other citrus fruits, are the best sources of vitamin C. Vitamin C is highly labile and is destroyed by several factors including heat, light and oxygen. A diet containing a diversity of plant foods, eaten either raw or lightly cooked, is therefore recommended. Foods such as stews, soups, jams and compotes normally undergo prolonged cooking, which will significantly reduce and usually destroy all the vitamin C present.

Low intake
The vitamin C deficiency disease, scurvy, is uncommon in populations unless there is a prolonged shortage of fruit and vegetables together with an overall reduction in the food supply. Symptoms of deficiency such as weakness, fatigue, inflamed and bleeding gums, impaired wound healing and bruising have been observed after 3–6 months on a diet lacking vitamin C. The RNIs for preventing vitamin C deficiency are shown in Table 20.

Table 20. Recommended nutrient intakes for vitamin C in mg/day				
Age	United Kingdom	United States	European Union	WHO
0–3 months	25	30	–	20
4–6 months	25	30	–	20
7–9 months	25	35	20	20
10–12 months	25	35	20	20
1–3 years	30	40	25	20
4–6 years	30	45	25	20

Source: Garrow et al. (2).

High intake

Vitamin C is water-soluble and any excess is excreted in the urine. The toxicity of vitamin C is low and there is no risk to health of a high intake.

VITAMIN D

Function

Vitamin D has an active role in calcium and bone metabolism, stimulating the intestinal absorption of calcium and the release of bound calcium from the skeleton. In addition, vitamin D has a role in muscle function, in cell proliferation and maturation, and in the immune system. This may partly explain the susceptibility to anaemia and infection of children with rickets *(12,13)*.

Sources

Vitamin D is primarily synthesized in the skin by the action of ultraviolet B radiation from sunlight, after which it is further converted in the liver and kidneys to the active metabolite 1,25-dihydroxyvitamin D_3. Dietary vitamin D is obtained from fatty fish (sardines, salmon, herring, tuna, etc.), margarines (which in most countries are fortified with vitamin D), some dairy products (including infant formula), eggs, beef and liver. During complementary feeding, the amount of vitamin D obtained from the diet is generally low and exposure to daylight is thus important for infants and young children.

Requirements and RNIs

Because vitamin D is principally derived from the exposure of the skin to sunlight, establishing dietary recommendations (Table 21) is difficult.

The vitamin D status of the newborn is largely determined by the status of the mother. If maternal vitamin D status is poor during pregnancy, the newborn also has low plasma concentrations and low stores of vitamin D. The vitamin D content of breast-milk is also influenced by the vitamin D status of the mother, and because of the strong relationship between maternal and infant vitamin D status, in some countries vitamin D supplements are recommended for pregnant women.

Children under 3 years of age are particularly vulnerable to poor vitamin D status because of the high demands of growth and the rapid rate at which calcium is laid down in bone. However, the amount of sunlight exposure needed to achieve the vitamin D requirements of infants is not large. Exposure of the face alone (or of the lower arms or legs) to sunlight for around

Age	United Kingdom	United States[a]	European Union	WHO
0–3 months	8.5	7.5	10–25	10
4–6 months	8.5	7.5	10–25	10
7–9 months	7.0	10	10	10
10–12 months	7.0	10	10	10
1–3 years	7.0	10	10	10
4–6 years	0[b]	10	0–10	10

Table 21. Recommended nutrient intakes for vitamin D in µg/day

[a] According to the US Institute of Medicine (15) an adequate intake for the whole period (0–6 years) is 5 µg/day.

[b] If exposed to the sun.

Source: Garrow et al. (2).

30 minutes each day is calculated to yield around 10 µg (400 IU) vitamin D per day, an amount similar to the RNI for young children. Because it is fat-soluble, enough vitamin D can be stored to supply the physiological requirements over days or even months when there is no sun.

The ability to synthesize vitamin D from sunlight varies according to location and time of year. Those who live at a southerly latitude in the Region can synthesize sufficient vitamin D from a minimal amount of sun exposure from April through to October, with very reduced or no synthesis during the remaining part of the year. During the northern winters there may be 6 or more months of very little or no sun, so that infants and young children in the north may require vitamin D supplements during this time.

Infants should not be placed in direct sunlight for long periods because of the risk of sunburn, especially around midday in the summer. Sun-screen creams should prevent sunburn in countries with extreme heat and long hours of sunshine. However, sun-screens can reduce or even stop the synthesis of vitamin D, and around 15 minutes of exposure without sunscreen in the early morning or late afternoon when the sun is less damaging is therefore recommended. Within the WHO European Region, because of the wide variation in latitudes, the policies needed to prevent vitamin D deficiency will vary markedly.

Some European countries recommend that infants receive a daily supplement of vitamin D. In the United Kingdom, for example, it is recommended that breastfed infants aged 6 months or more and pregnant and lactating women be given supplements of 7 µg/day. In most countries where there are recommendations for vitamin D supplementation, doses of 7–10 µg (280–400 IU)/ day are usually recommended. There is still doubt, however, about how much should be given to lactating mothers deficient in vitamin D to ensure optimum levels of the vitamin in breast-milk. In a population in Finland with scant sunlight in winter, breastfeeding by mothers who received as much as 25 µg (1000 IU)/day was not sufficient to secure adequate vitamin D status in their infants *(14)*.

Low intake

Infants at risk of vitamin D deficiency are those whose skin is completely covered, who are dark-skinned, who live in northern latitudes or who are weaned on to vegan diets. Growth failure, lethargy and irritability are early signs of deficiency. Prolonged vitamin D deficiency in infants and young children results in rickets, which occurs only when bones are still growing. In rickets, there is a reduced calcification of the growing ends (epiphyses) of the bones. The clinical manifestations of rickets vary with age and with the duration of vitamin D deficiency. As the disease progresses, the epiphysis of the long bones and the ribs tend to be most seriously affected, resulting in flaring of the wrists and ankles, beading of the rib cage and softening of the skull bones (craniotabes). Some information on the prevalence of rickets in the WHO European Region is given in Chapter 1 (see page 26).

Rickets usually occurs in young children owing to their high rate of growth. The situation is aggravated by factors such as the tradition of swaddling (completely covering infants), keeping infants indoors or keeping them completely covered when out of doors. Swaddling, which reduces exposure of the skin to sun, still occurs in many parts of the Region and should certainly be discouraged. Infants should not be completely covered, and children should play out of doors as much as possible. Preventive measures for pregnant women and children under 5 years, such as dietary education and behavioural interventions, should be implemented. Where rickets is a public health problem, all infants should receive a vitamin D supplement in addition to adequate sunlight.

High intake

High intakes of vitamin D can be toxic at all ages and infants are especially vulnerable. Hypercalcaemia (raised plasma concentrations of calcium) arising from vitamin D intakes of 50 µg/day or more has been reported. Hypercalcaemia is associated with thirst, anorexia, failure to thrive, vomiting, depressed IQ, raised plasma levels of vitamin D, and the risk of calcification of soft tissues and the formation of calcium stones in the renal tract.

REFERENCES

1. UNDERWOOD, B.A. Maternal vitamin A status and its importance in infancy and early childhood. *American journal of clinical nutrition,* 52 (Suppl. 2): S175–S225 (1994).

2. GARROW, J.S. ET AL., ED. *Human nutrition and dietetics,* 10th ed. London, Churchill Livingstone, 1999.

3. MORSE, C. *The prevalence and causes of anemia in Muynak District, Karakalpakistan, the Republic of Uzbekistan.* Brandon, MS, Crosslink International, 1994.

4. BRANCA, F. ET AL. *The health and nutritional status of children and women in Armenia.* Rome, National Institute of Nutrition, 1998.

5. BRANCA, F. ET AL. *Mulitiple indicator cluster survey in Fyrom with micronutrient component.* Rome, National Institute of Nutrition, 1999.

6. KEUSCH, G.T. Vitamin A supplements – too good not to be true. *New England journal of medicine,* 323: 985–987 (1990).

7. FILTEAU, S.M. & TOMKINS, A.M. Vitamin A supplementation in developing countries. *Archives of disease in childhood,* 72: 106–109 (1995).

8. INTERNATIONAL VITAMIN A CONSULTATIVE GROUP. *IVACG statement: vitamin A and iron interactions.* Washington, DC, Nutrition Foundation, 1996.

9. DEPARTMENT OF HEALTH, UNITED KINGDOM. *Dietary reference values for food energy and nutrients for the United Kingdom. Report of the Panel on Dietary Reference Values of the Committee on Medical Aspects of Food Policy.* London, H.M. Stationery Office, 1991 (Report on Health and Social Subjects, No. 41).

10. FOMON, S.J. & OLSON, J.A. Vitamin A and the carotenoids. *In:* Fomon, S.J. *Nutrition of normal infants.* St Louis, MO, Mosby, 1993.

11. ALLEN, L.H. & AHLUWALIA, N. *Improving iron status through diet: the application of knowledge concerning dietary iron availability in human populations.* Washington, DC, US Agency for International Development, 1997.

12. GRINDULIS, H. ET AL. Combined deficiency of iron and vitamin D in Asian toddlers. *Archives of disease in childhood,* 61: 843–848 (1986).

13. LAWSON, M. & THOMAS, M. Vitamin D concentration in Asian children aged 2 years living in England: population survey. *British medical journal,* 318: 28 (1999).

14. ALA-HOUHALA, M. 25-Hydroxyvitamin D levels during breastfeeding with or without maternal or infantile supplementation of vitamin D. *Journal of pediatric gastroenterology and nutrition*, 4: 220–226 (1985).
15. US INSTITUTE OF MEDICINE. *Dietary reference intakes for calcium, phosphorus, magnesium, vitamin D, and fluoride*. Washington, DC, National Academy Press, 1997.

Appendix

Recommended nutrient intakes for vitamins not discussed in this chapter (from Garrow et al. *(2)*)

Vitamin E (mg α–tocopherol/day)

Age	United Kingdom	United States	European Union	WHO
0–3 months	0.4 mg/g PUFA[a]	3	0.4 mg/g PUFA	0.15–2 mg/kg body weight
4–6 months	0.4 mg/g PUFA	3	0.4 mg/g PUFA	0.15–2 mg/kg body weight
7–9 months	0.4 mg/g PUFA	4	0.4 mg/g PUFA	0.15–2 mg/kg body weight
10–12 months	0.4 mg/g PUFA	4	0.4 mg/g PUFA	0.15–2 mg/kg body weight
1–3 years	0.4 mg/g PUFA	6	0.4 mg/g PUFA	0.15–2 mg/kg body weight
4–6 years	–	7	–	0.15–2 mg/kg body weight

[a] PUFA = polyunsaturated fatty acid.

Vitamin K (µg/day)

Age	United Kingdom	United States	European Union	WHO
0–3 months	10	5	–	–
4–6 months	10	5	–	–
7–9 months	10	10	–	–
10–12 months	10	10	–	–
1–3 years	–	15	–	–
4–6 years	–	20	–	–

Vitamin B$_1$ (thiamin)

Age	United Kingdom		United States	European Union	WHO
	mg/day	mg/1000 kcal	mg/day	mg/day	mg/day
0–3 months	0.2	0.3	0.3	–	0.3
4–6 months	0.2	0.3	0.3	–	0.3
7–9 months	0.3	0.3	0.4	0.3	0.3
10–12 months	0.3	0.3	0.4	0.3	0.3
1–3 years	0.5	0.4	0.7	0.5	0.5
4–6 years	0.7	0.4	0.9	0.7	0.7

Vitamin B$_2$ (riboflavin) (mg/day)

Age	United Kingdom	United States	European Union	WHO
0–3 months	0.4	0.4	–	0.5
4–6 months	0.4	0.4	–	0.5
7–9 months	0.4	0.5	0.4	0.5
10–12 months	0.4	0.5	0.4	0.5
1–3 years	0.6	0.8	0.8	0.8
4–6 years	0.8	1.1	1.0	1.1

Vitamin B$_3$ (niacin or nicotinic acid)

Age	United Kingdom[a]	United States	European Union[b]	WHO
	mg/day	mg/day	mg/day	mg/day
0–3 months	3	5	–	5.4
4–6 months	3	5	–	5.4
7–9 months	5	6	5	5.4
10–12 months	5	6	5	5.4
1–3 years	8	9	9	9.0
4–6 years	11	12	11	12.1

[a] 6.6 mg/1000 kcal.
[b] 1.6 mg/MJ.

Vitamin B$_6$ (pyridoxine)

Age	United Kingdom		United States	European Union[a]	WHO
	mg/day	µg/g protein	mg/day	mg/day	
0–3 months	0.2	8	0.3	–	–
4–6 months	0.2	8	0.3	–	–
7–9 months	0.3	10	0.6	0.4	–
10–12 months	0.4	13	0.6	0.4	–
1–3 years	0.7	13	1.0	0.7	–
4–6 years	0.9	13	1.1	0.9	–

[a] 15 µg/g protein.

Biotin (µg/day)

Age	United Kingdom	United States	European Union	WHO
0–3 months	–	10	–	–
4–6 months	–	10	–	–
7–9 months	–	15	–	–
10–12 months	–	15	–	–
1–3 years	–	20	–	–
4–6 years	–	25–30	–	–

Pantothenic acid (mg/day)

Age	United Kingdom	United States	European Union	WHO
0–3 months	1.7	2.0	–	–
4–6 months	1.7	2.0	–	–
7–9 months	1.7	3.0	–	–
10–12 months	1.7	3.0	–	–
1–3 years	1.7	3.0	–	–
4–6 years	3–7	3–5	–	–

CHAPTER 5

Minerals other than iron

In countries where iodine deficiency is a public health problem, legislation on universal salt iodization should be adopted and enforced.

Many minerals are essential micronutrients and play a vital role in growth, health and development. Those that are most important in the complementary feeding of infants and young children, namely iodine, zinc, calcium and sodium, are discussed here. The RNIs of those minerals that are not discussed (phosphorus, magnesium, potassium, chloride, copper and selenium) are given in the Appendix to this chapter. Table 22 lists the main sources and functions of a number of minerals.

IODINE

Function

Iodine is an essential substrate in the synthesis of the thyroid hormones, which are among the key regulators of metabolism *(1)*. The thyroid hormones are required for normal growth and development, for oxygen consumption in cells, and for the maintenance of metabolic rate *(2)*. Thyroid hormones are also important in mental development and mental retardation, and congenital deafness can be due to hypothyroidism induced by iodine deficiency *in utero (3)*. It is therefore important that both maternal stores and the maternal diet during pregnancy contain adequate quantities of iodine.

Sources

The iodine content of plants and animals is determined by the environment in which they live and grow. Iodine deficiency is especially prevalent in mountainous regions, but can also occur at sites of prior glaciation and in low-lying areas subject to flooding. As most soils contain little iodine, most foodstuffs are poor sources and food grown in iodine-deficient regions cannot provide enough iodine for the population or livestock living there *(4)*.

Fruits, vegetables, cereals, meat and meat products contain between 20 and 50 μg iodine/kg under normal circumstances. The only naturally rich source of iodine is sea fish (160–1400 μg/kg). Around 200 g of sea fish, eaten weekly, should provide young children with an intake equal to around

Table 22. The main sources and functions of minerals

Mineral	Important sources	Functions
Iron	Liver, meat, poultry, egg yolk, sardines, mackerel, whole grain cereals and breads, legumes, spinach	Component of red blood cell pigment Component of muscle
Calcium	Milk, cheese, shrimps, salmon, sardines, herring, green leafy vegetables	Growth of bones and teeth Contraction of muscles Nerve transmission
Zinc	Meat, fish, eggs, cereals, legumes	Growth Reproduction Wound healing
Iodine	Iodized salt, seafood, animal and plant foods grown in non-goitrogenic coastal areas	Formation of thyroid hormone
Fluoride	Fluoridated water, tea, seafood, infant foods made with bone meal	Hardening of teeth and bones
Magnesium	Roasted peanuts, dry beans, raw spinach and other green vegetables	Nerve and muscle activity Important for many enzyme reactions
Sodium	Salt, meat, fish, eggs, milk	Essential in the control of extracellular volume and acid-base balance, cellular electrical activity, nerve conduction and muscle function
Phosphorus	Milk, cheese, shrimps, salmon, sardines, herring, green leafy vegetables	Bone metabolism
Potassium	Fruit and vegetables	Maintenance of electrolyte balance
Copper	Shellfish, legumes, whole grain cereals, liver	Cofactor in metalloenzymes
Selenium	Cereal grains, meat, fish	Cofactor in antioxidants

50 μg iodine per day *(5)*. In the United Kingdom *(6)* and some Nordic countries, milk and dairy products are the main source of iodine because cattle fodder is iodized by law. Seasonal variations are seen, and in Nordic countries around 45% and 70% of total iodine intake in summer and winter, respectively, comes from cow's milk and milk products.

Requirements and RNIs

Iodine is readily absorbed and excess intake is well controlled by renal excretion. In the presence of goitrogens (found in cabbage, turnips, swedes, brussels sprouts and broccoli, for example) the utilization of absorbed iodine is decreased and therefore iodine intake should be increased. The RNIs for iodine (Table 23) are based on the requirement for the prevention of goitre (about 1–2 μg/kg body weight) plus a 100% safety margin.

Table 23. Recommended nutrient intakes for iodine in μg/day				
Age	United Kingdom	United States	European Union	WHO
0–3 months	50	40	–	40
4–6 months	60	40	–	40
7–9 months	60	50	50	50
10–12 months	60	50	50	50
1–3 years	70	70	70	70–120
4–6 years	100	100	90	70–120

Sources: World Health Organization *(7)*; Garrow et al. *(8)*.

In European countries with mild iodine deficiency, the recommendation has been made to extend the RNI of 90 μg/day down to 0–12 months because such an intake is required to achieve positive iodine balance in the growing infant *(9)*. In populations where there is no evidence of widespread iodine deficiency disorders, exclusive breastfeeding for the first few months will supply infants with the iodine required.

Low intake

Iodine deficiency is the world's greatest single cause of preventable brain damage and mental retardation *(3)*. The term "iodine deficiency disorders" refers to the wide spectrum of effects of iodine deficiency on growth and development. The deficiency results in a reduced synthesis of thyroid hormone. In an attempt to sequester more iodine, the thyroid gland enlarges leading to goitre, which is the most obvious and familiar sign of iodine deficiency. Other effects are seen at all stages of development, however, and are particularly pertinent during the fetal and neonatal periods (Table 24).

Table 24. Effects of iodine deficiency during early development	
Stage of development	**Disorder**
Fetus	Abortion and stillbirth
	Congenital abnormalities
	Deafness
	Increased perinatal mortality
	Increased infant mortality
	Neurological cretinism
	Myxoedematous cretinism
	Psychomotor defects
Neonate	Neonatal goitre
	Neonatal hypothyroidism
Child	Goitre
	Juvenile hypothyroidism
	Impaired mental function
	Retarded physical development

Source: Hetzel *(10)*.

In populations where iodine deficiency disorders are widespread and severe enough to induce hypothyroxinaemia during gestation, the physiological transfer of thyroid hormones from the mother to the fetus is decreased. The consequence is irreversible brain damage manifest in the neurological features of endemic cretinism. Moreover, iodine deficiency occurring during late gestation and persisting during lactation leads to a low iodine content of breast-milk and possible perinatally acquired hypothyroidism in the breastfed infant. This explains the hypothyroid component of endemic cretinism *(11)*.

In regions with endemic iodine deficiency disorders, prevention of both brain damage and hypothyroidism in the breastfed infant requires iodine supplementation starting early in gestation, or preferably before conception, and extending throughout lactation *(11)*. Lower breast-milk iodine concentrations have been reported in endemic iodine-deficient areas *(12)*.

Iodine deficiency increases the sensitivity of children to the carcinogenic effect of thyroid radiation. The exposure to radioactive fallout around Chernobyl is thought to have played a major role in the development of hypothyroidism and thyroid cancer in the exposed population *(13)*.

Correction of iodine deficiency disorders

Because iodine deficiency results mainly from geological rather than social and economic conditions, it cannot be eliminated by changes in dietary habits. The solution to iodine deficiency has focused on two main strategies, iodine supplementation and iodine fortification. Universal salt iodization, calling for household salt and all salt used in agriculture, food processing/manufacturing and catering to be iodized, is the agreed prevention strategy *(14)*.

The choice of this approach has been based on the following facts *(15)*.

- Salt is one of the few commodities that comes closest to being universally consumed.
- Salt consumption is almost stable throughout the year in a given region.
- Salt production is usually limited to a few centres.
- Salt iodization technology is available at reasonable cost (0.4–1.5 US cents per kilogram and 2–8 US cents per person per year).
- The addition of iodine to salt does not affect its colour, taste or odour.
- The quality of iodized salt can be monitored at production, retail and household levels.

Other vehicles for iodine fortification include bread, milk, water and other foods. Occasional successes have been reported when using them *(6,16)*. Nevertheless, universal salt iodization remains the strategy of choice. The intake of other vehicles (except water) is not essential for survival, and they are frequently not consumed by those most vulnerable such as pregnant women, children and poor and isolated populations.

National universal salt iodization programmes should be implemented through legislation and should take into account locally produced and imported salt. Care should be taken to ensure that the promotion of iodized salt does not result in an increase in salt intake. The necessary monitoring of iodized salt intake is a unique opportunity to evaluate and monitor salt intake and to respect and support the WHO recommendation to maintain salt intake at healthy levels. In particular, iodized salt is not appropriate for infants and young children because of their limited ability to excrete sodium (see Chapter 8 and page 95). Their requirement for iodine will be met if salt is universally iodized, because both breast-milk and formula milk will then have an adequate content of iodine. Complementary foods of animal origin, notably fish given at around 6 months of age and cow's milk and milk products after 9 months of age, can also provide sufficient iodine.

As an interim measure until an effective universal iodized salt system is fully operational, iodine supplementation can be considered in endemic regions to immediately prevent the adverse effects of iodine deficiency on the central nervous system. Such measures should not delay or compromise the implementation of the agreed strategy of universal salt iodization. The recommendations for supplementation are as follows.

- Where mild to moderate iodine deficiency disorders exist, pregnant and lactating women should be given iodine supplements until their iodine intake reaches 200–300 µg/day. Infants and children should be given the physiological dose of 90 µg/day up to the age of 3 years, by which time most brain development has occurred.

- In conditions of severe iodine deficiency (goitre prevalence ≥ 30% and median urinary iodine below 20 µg/l), and especially if neonatal hypothyroidism and cretinism continue to occur, the administration of iodized oil to women of child-bearing age is justified, ideally before pregnancy. This procedure is efficient and safe *(17)*.

- In all conditions of iodine deficiency, if infant formula is used it should contain 10 µg iodine/dl for full-term infants and 20 µg/dl for preterm infants.

High intake
Any unnecessarily high intake of iodine is excreted in the urine. Nevertheless, excessive iodine intake at the population level can have adverse effects *(18)*. The most important is the development of hyperthyroidism in adults with nodular goitre. Other possible complications include iodine-induced autoimmune thyroid disorders and a change in the predominant type of thyroid cancer. In infants and children, the main complication of iodine excess is iodine-induced hypothyroidism *(19)*. Susceptibility to the side effects of excess iodine depends on the baseline iodine intake before

exposure to excess *(20)*. In conditions of normal iodine intake, the upper limit for adults is considered to be 1000 µg/day, and for 0–8-year-olds probably 300 µg/day.

ZINC

Function
Because zinc is a constituent of many enzymes in the body, it is important in a wide range of metabolic processes including protein and nucleic acid synthesis. Zinc is mainly absorbed in the duodenum. Its main route of excretion is through the gastrointestinal tract and, to a lesser extent, via the kidneys and the skin.

Sources
In general, zinc from animal products is better absorbed than that from plant foods. Good sources of zinc include red meat, liver, seafoods, milk and dairy products, pulses, wheat and rice. Unrefined cereal grains and legumes are rich in phytate, which reduces zinc absorption. In addition, zinc absorption can be limited by the intake of phosphates and calcium, and supplementation with large doses of non-haem iron can also reduce its bioavailability. In contrast, haem iron has no effect on zinc bioavailability. Zinc absorption is enhanced by a number of dietary factors including amino acids (particularly histidine), lactose and a low level of dietary iron.

Requirements and RNIs
Requirements for dietary zinc are determined partly by the physiological processes governing tissue demands for zinc and its rate of loss from the body, and partly by the intrinsic characteristics of the diet. Requirements are markedly increased during periods of "catch-up growth", when infants and young children are recovering from malnutrition or infection.

Breast-milk is fully adequate to meet the infant's basal requirements for zinc up to 6 months of age. Infants absorb up to about 80% of the zinc in breast-milk compared to 30% from cow's milk formula and about 15% from soya-based formula. Estimates of infant zinc requirements between the ages of 6 and 12 months, however, suggest that the declining daily output of zinc in milk will be insufficient if breast-milk is the sole source. It is thus particularly desirable to select diets with a high zinc bioavailability for infants after 6 months of age.

The RNIs for zinc are shown in Table 25.

Table 25. Recommended nutrient intakes for zinc in mg/day				
Age	United Kingdom	United States	European Union	WHO[a]
0–3 months	4.0	5.0	–	5.3
4–6 months	4.0	5.0	–	3.1
7–9 months	5.0	5.0	4.0	5.6
10–12 months	5.0	5.0	4.0	5.6
1–3 years	5.0	10.0	4.0	5.5
4–6 years	6.5	10.0	6.0	6.5

[a] Normative requirement on diet of moderate zinc availability.

Source: Garrow et al. *(8)*.

Low intake

Zinc deficiency is primarily caused by a diet low in animal products and high in phytate, or as a result of high zinc losses due to diarrhoea. The clinical features of zinc deficiency are diverse and nonspecific (growth retardation, for example) unless the deficiency is very severe. Acrodermatitis enteropathica is a genetic defect that results in failure of zinc absorption and is thus not a "nutritional" disorder *(21)*. Manifestations of zinc deficiency are similar, however, and include skin lesions, impaired wound healing, impaired taste, depressed appetite, diarrhoea and defects of the immune system, the latter resulting in an increased susceptibility to infections *(7)*.

The effects of marginal or mild zinc deficiency are less obvious and can easily be overlooked. A slowed growth rate and impaired resistance to infection are frequently the only manifestations of mild deficiency in humans *(7)*.

Investigations into the impact of zinc supplements on the growth of infants and young children in developing countries have shown inconsistent results. In situations where physical growth is compromised, however, zinc supplementation appears to have a positive impact on children's growth *(22)*. Furthermore, it has been suggested that maternal supplementation with zinc improves certain pregnancy outcomes such as birth weight and head circumference *(23)*.

High intake

Few instances of acute zinc poisoning have been reported. Its manifestations include nausea, vomiting, diarrhoea, fever and lethargy and have been observed after ingestion of 4–8 g of zinc. Long-term exposure to high zinc intakes substantially in excess of requirements has been shown to interfere with the metabolism of other trace elements, mainly copper (7).

CALCIUM

Function
Calcium is essential for the structural integrity and mineralization of bones and teeth and plays an important role in a number of metabolic and regulatory processes. It is a cofactor of many enzymes necessary for nerve and muscle function, a component of the blood clotting cascade and a regulator of many intracellular processes. An adequate supply of calcium is vital during skeletal growth to ensure optimum bone mass.

Sources
Milk and milk products provide the richest and most easily absorbed dietary sources of calcium. Other good sources include nuts and fish. Components binding calcium, such as phosphorus, phytate and oxalate can reduce its bioavailability.

Requirements and RNIs
Breast-milk contains a high level of calcium and is sufficient to meet the infant's requirements up to about 6 months. After this, breast-milk should continue to provide most of the calcium needed by infants and young children. Recommended calcium intakes are shown in Table 26.

Low intake
Isolated calcium deficiency rarely occurs in childhood. In practice, this only happens in young children who receive no milk or dairy products. The disturbances in calcium metabolism associated with rickets and steatorrhoea are

Table 26. Recommended nutrient intakes for calcium in mg/day				
Age	United Kingdom	United States	European Union	WHO
0–3 months	525	210	–	500
4–6 months	525	210	–	500
7–9 months	525	270	400	600
10–12 months	525	270	400	600
1–3 years	350	500	400	400
4–6 years	450	800	450	450

Source: Garrow et al. (8).

usually related to vitamin D deficiency rather than to calcium, although rickets resulting from deficiency in calcium has been described *(24)*. The calcium intake of infants fed macrobiotic diets may be less than half that of infants fed nonvegetarian or lactovegetarian diets, and high concentrations of phytates and oxalates may further reduce calcium absorption from macrobiotic diets. Very low calcium intake in children may result in rickets, growth retardation and biochemical signs of hyperparathyroidism *(24)*.

Calcium absorption may be impaired through binding with long-chain fatty acids present in formula milks and unmodified cow's milk. Hypocalcaemia may cause seizures and tetany (musculoskeletal spasms and twitching, particularly in the fingers and face) and tingling and numbness. Feeding modified, low-phosphorus infant formula to non-breastfed infants has virtually eliminated the problem.

If infants and young children are fed a diet with no breast-milk, cow's milk or milk products (after 9 months), it is almost impossible to reach the RNI for calcium. As a result, it is common to recommend that such infants and children receive a daily calcium supplement. However, the long-term consequences of a calcium intake below the RNI are not known for this age group.

High intake
There is little evidence that excessive intake of calcium will result in harm apart from the extreme situation of "milk-alkali" syndrome, which rarely occurs in childhood *(21)*. Ingestion of large amounts of alkaline calcium salts can override the ability of the kidneys to excrete unwanted calcium, causing hypercalcaemia and metastatic calcification of the cornea, kidneys and blood vessels. Hypercalcaemia (high blood calcium) results in thirst, mild mental confusion and irritability, loss of appetite, fatigue and weakness.

SODIUM
Function
The majority of sodium is found in extracellular fluids. It is essential in the control of extracellular volume and acid–base balance, cellular electrical activity, nerve conduction and muscle function.

Sources
The sodium content of naturally occurring foods is relatively low, with small amounts in meat, fish, eggs and milk. Most dietary sodium is provided as salt. Some salt is added in cooking and at the table, but in many countries of the WHO European Region the largest proportion (around 80%)

is obtained from processed foods, to which salt and other sodium-containing compounds are added during manufacturing. Especially high amounts of sodium are found in sausages, bread, ham, pickles and sauces (see Chapter 8).

Low intake

Infants are efficient at conserving sodium by regulating losses in the urine. In general, there is little risk of becoming sodium-deficient. Rapid and excessive losses during sweating because of extreme temperatures, or in severe gastrointestinal diseases with losses through diarrhoea and vomiting, may lead to symptoms of sodium depletion and necessitate a temporary increase in sodium intake.

High intake

Infants are less efficient than adults at excreting excess sodium, and the sodium intakes of infants should therefore be moderated. By about 4 months, healthy infants can begin to excrete an excessive sodium load. However, complementary foods should contain only very small amounts of salt. This can be achieved by not adding salt to foods and by avoiding highly salted foods such as pickled and highly processed, smoked and cured foods.

In infants, hypernatraemia (high blood sodium concentration) is usually associated with excessive sodium intake from inappropriately composed feeds, and dehydration due to net loss of water in excess of net loss of sodium. In severe hypernatraemic dehydration, the renal ability to excrete sodium becomes impaired, thus exacerbating the problem (25).

Recommended sodium intakes are given in Table 27.

Table 27. Recommended nutrient intakes for sodium in mg/day				
Age	United Kingdom	United States	European Union[a]	WHO
0–3 months	210	120	–	–
4–6 months	280	120	–	–
7–9 months	320	200	–	–
10–12 months	350	200	–	–
1–3 years	500	225	–	–
4–6 years	700	300	575–3500	–

[a] Acceptable range.

Source: Garrow et al. (8).

REFERENCES

1. TAUROG, A. Hormone synthesis: thyroid iodine metabolism. *In*: Braverman, L.E. & Utiger, R.D., ed. *Werner & Ingbar's the thyroid.* Hagerstown, MD, Lippincott Williams & Wilkins, 2000, pp. 47–81.
2. BERNAL, J. & NUNEZ, J. Thyroid hormones and brain development. *European journal of endocrinology,* **133**: 390–398 (1995).
3. STANBURY, J.B. *The damaged brain of iodine deficiency: cognitive, behavioral, neuromotor, educative aspects.* New York, Cognizant Communication, 1993.
4. KOUTRAS, D.A. ET AL. The ecology of iodine. *In*: Stanbury, J.B. & Hetzel, B.S., ed. *Endemic goiter and endemic cretinism.* New York, John Wiley, 1980, pp. 185–195.
5. WAYNE, E.J. ET AL. *Clinical aspects of iodine metabolism.* Oxford, Blackwell, 1964.
6. PHILLIPS, D.I.W. Iodine, milk, and the elimination of endemic goitre in Britain: the story of an accidental public health triumph. *Journal of epidemiology and community health,* **51**: 391–393(1997).
7. *Trace elements in human nutrition and health.* Geneva, World Health Organization, 1996.
8. GARROW, J.S. ET AL., ED. *Human nutrition and dietetics,* 10th ed. London, Churchill Livingstone, 1999.
9. DELANGE, F. Requirements of iodine in humans. *In*: Delange, F. et al., ed. *Iodine deficiency in Europe. A continuing concern.* New York, Plenum Press, 1993, pp. 5–16.
10. HETZEL, B.S. Iodine deficiency disorders (IDD) and their eradication. *Lancet,* **2**: 1126–1129 (1983).
11. DELANGE, F. Endemic cretinism. *In*: Braverman, L.E. & Utiger, R.D., ed. *Werner & Ingbar's the thyroid.* Hagerstown, MD, Lippincott Williams & Wilkins, 2000, pp. 744–754.
12. DELANGE, F. ET AL. Physiopathology of iodine nutrition during pregnancy, lactation and early postnatal life. *In*: Berger, H., ed. *Vitamins and minerals in pregnancy and lactation.* New York, Raven Press, 1988, pp. 205–213.
13. WILLIAMS, E.D. The role of iodine deficiency in radiation induced thyroid cancer. *In*: Delange, F. et al., ed. *Elimination of iodine deficiency disorders (IDD) in central and eastern Europe, the Commonwealth of Independent States and the Baltic states. Proceedings of a conference held in Munich, Germany, 3–6 September 1997.* Copenhagen, WHO Regional Office for Europe, 1998 (document WHO/EURO/NUT/98.1), pp. 73–81.
14. *Indicators for assessing iodine deficiency disorders and their control through salt iodization.* Geneva, World Health Organization, 1994 (document WHO/NUT/94.6).

15. MANNAR, V.M.G. The iodization of salt for the elimination of iodine deficiency disorders. *In*: Hetzel, B.S. & Pandav, C.S., ed. *S.O.S. for a billion. The conquest of iodine deficiency disorders.* New Delhi, Oxford University Press, 1994, pp. 89–107.

16. DUNN, J.T. The use of iodized oil and other alternatives for the elimination of iodine deficiency disorders. *In*: Hetzel, B.S. & Pandav, C.S., ed. *S.O.S. for a billion. The conquest of iodine deficiency disorders.* New Delhi, Oxford University Press, 1994, pp. 119–128.

17. DELANGE, F. Administration of iodized oil during pregnancy: a summary of the published evidence. *Bulletin of the World Health Organization,* 74: 101–108 (1996).

18. DELANGE, F. & LECOMTE, P. Iodine supplementation: benefits outweigh risks. *Drug safety,* 22: 89–95 (2000).

19. DELANGE, F. ET AL. Topical iodine, breastfeeding and neonatal hypothyroidism. *Archives of disease in childhood,* 63: 102–107 (1988).

20. DELANGE, F. ET AL. Risks of iodine-induced hyperthyroidism following correction of iodine deficiency by iodized salt. *Thyroid,* 9: 545–556 (1999).

21. BARLTROP, D. Mineral deficiency. *In*: Campbell, A.G.M. et al., ed. *Forfar & Arneil's Textbook of Paediatrics,* 5th ed. Edinburgh, Churchill Livingstone, 1992.

22. *Complementary feeding of young children in developing countries: a review of current scientific knowledge.* Geneva, World Health Organization, 1998 (document WHO/NUT/98.1).

23. SAMMAN, S. Zinc. *In*: Mann, J. & Truswell, S., ed. *Essentials in human nutrition.* Oxford, Oxford University Press, 1998, pp. 151–157.

24. THACHER, T.D. ET AL. A comparison of calcium, vitamin D or both, for nutritional rickets in Nigerian children. *New England journal of medicine,* 341: 563–568 (1999).

25. FOMON, S.J. Sodium, chloride, and potassium. *In*: Fomon, S.J. *Nutrition of normal infants.* St Louis, MO, Mosby, 1993.

Appendix

Recommended nutrient intakes for minerals not discussed in this chapter (from Garrow et al. *(8)*)

Phosphorus (mg/day)

Age	United Kingdom	United States	European Union	WHO
0–3 months	400	–	–	–
4–6 months	400	–	–	–
7–9 months	400	–	300	–
10–12 months	400	–	300	–
1–3 years	270	460	300	–
4–6 years	350	500	350–450	–

Magnesium (mg/day)

Age	United Kingdom	United States	European Union	WHO
0–3 months	55	40	–	–
4–6 months	60	40	–	–
7–9 months	75	60	–	–
10–12 months	80	60	–	–
1–3 years	85	80	–	–
4–6 years	120	120	–	–

Potassium (mg/day)

Age	United Kingdom	United States (minumum) requirement)[a]	European Union	WHO
0–3 months	800	500	–	–
4–6 months	850	500	–	–
7–9 months	700	700	800	–
10–12 months	700	700	800	–
1–3 years	800	1000	800	–
4–6 years	1100	1400	1100	–

[a] Desirable intakes may exceed these values.

Chloride (mg/day)

Age	United Kingdom	United States (minumum) requirement)[a]	European Union	WHO
0–3 months	320	180	–	–
4–6 months	400	300	–	–
7–9 months	500	300	–	–
10–12 months	500	300	–	–
1–3 years	800	350	–	–
4–6 years	1100	500	–	–

[a] No allowance for large losses from the skin through sweat.

Copper (mg/day)

Age	United Kingdom	United States[a]	European Union	WHO[b]
0–3 months	0.3	0.4–0.6	–	0.33–0.55
4–6 months	0.3	0.4–0.6	–	0.37–0.62
7–9 months	0.3	0.6–0.7	0.3	0.6
10–12 months	0.3	0.6–0.7	0.3	0.6
1–3 years	0.4	0.7–1.0	0.4	0.56
4–6 years	0.6	1.0–1.5	0.6	0.57

[a] Upper levels should not be habitually exceeded because of toxicity.

[b] Normative requirement.

Selenium (µg/day)

Age	United Kingdom	United States	European Union	WHO[a]
0–3 months	10	10	–	6
4–6 months	13	10	–	9
7–9 months	10	15	8	12
10–12 months	10	15	8	12
1–3 years	15	20	10	20
4–6 years	20	20	15	24

[a] Normative requirement.

Control of iron deficiency

Iron deficiency in infants and young children is widespread and has serious consequences for child health. Prevention of iron deficiency should therefore be given high priority.

When complementary foods are introduced at about 6 months of age, it is important that iron-rich foods such as liver, meat, fish and pulses or iron-fortified complementary foods are included.

The too-early introduction of unmodified cow's milk and milk products is an important nutritional risk factor for the development of iron deficiency anaemia. Unmodified cow's milk should not therefore be introduced as a drink until the age of 9 months and thereafter can be increased gradually.

Because of their inhibitory effect on iron absorption, all types of tea (black, green and herbal) and coffee should be avoided until 24 months of age. After this age, tea should be avoided at mealtimes.

Optimal iron stores at birth are important for the prevention of iron deficiency in the infant and young child. To help ensure good infant iron stores, the mother should eat an iron-rich diet during pregnancy. At birth the umbilical cord should not be clamped and ligated until it stops pulsating.

INTRODUCTION

Iron deficiency is one of the commonest nutritional deficiencies worldwide, estimated to affect more than three billion people. It ranges in severity from iron depletion, which causes no physiological impairment, to iron deficiency anaemia, and can affect mental and motor development. Children under the age of 3 years, pregnant women and women of child-bearing age are particularly susceptible to iron deficiency. It is estimated that 43% of the world's infants and children under the age of 4 years suffer from iron deficiency anaemia *(1)*. In some parts of Europe, especially in the central Asian republics and among Asian children in the United Kingdom, the prevalence of iron deficiency anaemia is high (see Chapter 1). Young children are especially vulnerable to the development of iron deficiency between the ages of 6 and 24 months. The increased nutritional needs resulting from rapid growth are combined with a diet that may be low in iron and vitamin C and high in unmodified cow's milk and other inhibitors of iron absorption. Dietary recommendations concerning iron are therefore of special importance during the period of complementary feeding. Recommendations for complementary feeding should be given high priority by health ministries, and should always form an integral part of population strategies to control iron deficiency. Prevention of iron deficiency in infants and young children is possible through the relatively simple dietary strategies described below.

Definition of iron deficiency

Iron depletion is a decrease in iron stores. There is no evidence of functional consequences but iron depletion represents a threshold below which further decreases result in functional impairment. When iron stores are depleted, haemoglobin synthesis is impaired and the haemoglobin level begins to fall. As the haemoglobin level of most people is usually within the normal range, iron depletion usually happens before the haemoglobin level has reached the statistically determined cut-off that defines anaemia (2).

Iron deficiency anaemia is defined as iron deficiency resulting in a haemoglobin level that falls below the statistically defined age- and sex-dependent cut-off limit (2). Haemoglobin and haematocrit cut-off points that define anaemia according to age and sex are shown in Table 28.

In practice, diagnosis is often based on haemoglobin values alone, and the prevalence of anaemia is expressed as the percentage of individuals with a haemoglobin value below a certain cut-off point. Anaemia can be caused by a number of other factors, including infection; if, however, values for haematocrit are also low, this strengthens the likelihood that the low

Table 28. Haemoglobin and haematocrit cut-off points used to define anaemia

Age or sex	Haemoglobin (g/dl)	Haematocrit (%)
6 months to 5 years	11.0	33
5–11 years	11.5	34
12–13 years	12.0	36
Non-pregnant women	12.0	36
Pregnant women	11.0	33
Men	13.0	39

Source: World Health Organization (1).

haemoglobin value is the result of iron deficiency. The severity of anaemia can be classified as mild, moderate or severe, depending on the haemoglobin value (Table 29).

Table 29. Classification of anaemia and corresponding haemoglobin levels	
Classification	Haemoglobin level (g/dl)
Severe	< 7
Moderate	< 10 (in children aged between 6 months and 5 years)
	< 9 (in infants less than 6 months)
Mild	10–11

Source: World Health Organization (1).

In addition to haemoglobin and haematocrit, there are a number of other tests used to assess iron status. The resources available will determine which tests are used. Of special interest is the measurement of serum ferritin levels, which provides an indication of iron stores in individuals whether or not they are anaemic. The main disadvantage of this test is that serum ferritin levels increase during illness, because serum ferritin is an acute-phase reactant. Thus, the use of serum ferritin levels can lead to an underestimation of the prevalence of iron deficiency in populations where infection is common. A ferritin value below 10 µg/l (3) or 12 µg/l (1) is generally accepted as an indication of iron depletion in children under 5 years.

It is possible to identify iron deficiency as a cause of anaemia by giving an iron supplement for 1–2 months. If the haemoglobin level increases by 1 g/dl or more, iron deficiency is a likely cause of the anaemia. If it does not, however, iron deficiency should not be ruled out because of the possibility of poor compliance or inconsistent ingestion and absorption of iron.

In infants and young children there are still uncertainties about the appropriate cut-off values for both haemoglobin and serum ferritin levels. Low levels of ferritin do not necessarily imply functional iron deficiency in infants. The evidence for using 10–12 µg ferritin per litre as a cut-off to define iron depletion is based on extrapolation from older age groups. In several studies from industrialized countries, including those in healthy infants receiving iron-fortified foods, a surprisingly high percentage of infants (20%–30%) had < 11 g haemoglobin per decilitre, suggesting that the cut-off value may be too high. These studies have instead recommended the use of values of 10.5 or 10.3 g/dl or lower to define anaemia in infants *(4–6)*.

Causes of anaemia other than iron deficiency

Anaemia can be caused by factors other than iron deficiency, and these can be classified as nutritional, environmental, infectious and hereditary factors.

- Nutritional anaemia can be caused by deficiency of other nutrients, such as vitamin A, folic acid, vitamin B_{12}, vitamin C, riboflavin and copper. There is an interaction between iron and vitamin A *(7)*. In several studies from societies where deficiencies of both vitamin A and iron are common, treatment with both micronutrients is more effective in correcting anaemia than giving iron alone, most likely because vitamin A deficiency impairs mobilization of iron stores.

- Even very small amounts of lead can impair haem synthesis and thus cause anaemia. There is also an interaction between lead intoxication and iron deficiency, because lead and iron share the same absorption pathway. Because iron absorption is enhanced during iron deficiency, there is a tendency for the absorption of lead, if present in the environment, to increase and thereby aggravate anaemia. Geophagia (the habit of eating soil) is associated with iron deficiency anaemia. It is not clear, however, if geophagia has a positive effect on iron status due to the iron content of the soil, or whether other substances in the soil, such as lead, reduce the absorption of dietary iron. Aplastic anaemia (reduced platelet and white cell counts as well as those of red cells) can be associated with excessive exposure to industrial or agricultural pollutants.

- Systemic infections and chronic inflammation can cause anaemia that is not related to iron deficiency. However, infectious diseases are typically more frequent in areas with a high prevalence of iron deficiency, and the anaemia associated with infections can thus be multifactorial. This is especially the case in diseases associated with blood loss, such as hookworm infestation, dysentery and schistosomiasis. There is some evidence that hookworm infestation may be a problem in some of the central Asian republics. The anaemia often seen in patients with malaria is caused by haemolysis and is therefore not necessarily associated with iron deficiency. People with malaria often have iron deficiency for other reasons, however, and this exacerbates the anaemia caused by haemolysis. As a result, malaria sufferers are often treated with iron in addition to antimalarials.

- Anaemia is also a sign of a number of hereditary haemoglobinopathies such as thalassaemia, sickle cell disease and glucose-6-phosphate dehydrogenase deficiency.

PHYSIOLOGY AND PATHOPHYSIOLOGY OF IRON

The largest pool of iron is present in the haemoglobin of red blood cells, which transport oxygen from the lungs to the tissues. The second largest pool is the myoglobin found in muscle, which stores the oxygen needed for muscle contraction. Storage iron located in the liver and the reticuloendothelial system represents the third major pool. An estimate of the size of these three pools in a 12-month-old infant is given in Fig. 14 (based on values taken from Fomon (8)).

Iron has several special characteristics that distinguish it from most other nutrients. Only a small fraction (around 10% or less) of the total iron in the diet is absorbed. Moreover, the body has no mechanisms specifically

Fig. 14. Iron balance and influencing factors in a 12-month-old infant

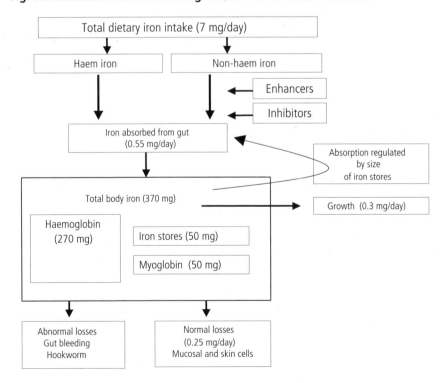

designed to excrete iron, and normal losses that occur through the gut or skin are very small. Regulation of total body iron therefore occurs through regulation of the absorption of iron.

Absorption

Haem and non-haem iron

There are two types of iron in food: haem iron and non-haem iron, and they are absorbed by different mechanisms. Haem iron is present in haemo-globin and myoglobin in meat (particularly liver) and fish, and is better absorbed than non-haem iron. The average absorption of haem iron from meat is around 25%. In contrast to non-haem iron, the absorption of haem iron is influenced very little by other constituents of the diet and by iron status. Nevertheless, most dietary iron is present in the form of non-haem iron. Complementary foods for infants may contain little meat and so most of the dietary iron is in the non-haem form. Absorption of non-haem iron is much lower than that of haem iron and depends on the iron status of the individual: more non-haem iron is absorbed by iron-deficient individuals and less by those who are iron-replete. Moreover, the absorption of non-haem iron depends on its solubility in the intestine, and this is determined by the composition of foods consumed in a meal. Vitamin C is a reducing agent and a potent promoter of iron absorption, increasing iron solubility through the oxidation of elemental iron from the ferrous (Fe^{2+}) to the ferric (Fe^{3+}) state to form a soluble compound. The promoters and inhibitors present in the diet are often stronger determinants of iron status than its actual iron content.

Promoters and inhibitors

The quantity of absorbed iron in the diet depends on the balance between the inhibitors and promoters (Table 30). Because the interaction takes place in the gastrointestinal tract, the inhibitory or enhancing effects of food components on non-haem iron absorption are greatest when these components are consumed in the same meal.

One of the strongest promoters of iron absorption is vitamin C in fresh vegetables and fruits, and there is a clear dose–response relationship between vitamin C intake and iron absorption (10). Fermented products such as kefir and sauerkraut also enhance non-haem iron absorption. In the presence of acid, complexes are formed with iron that prevent the formation of the less absorbable iron phytate. In addition, certain forms of milling and thermal processing reduce the phytate content of plant-based staples and thereby help to increase the absorption of non-haem iron. Mild

Table 30. Dietary compounds that inhibit (–) and enhance (+) the absorption of non-haem iron		
Food	**Degree of effect**	**Active substance**
Inhibiting		
Whole grain cereals and maize	– – –	Phytate
Tea, green leafy vegetables	– – –	Polyphenols
Milk, cheese	– –	Calcium plus phosphate
Spinach	–	Polyphenols, oxalic acid
Eggs	–	Phosphoprotein, albumin
Cereals	–	Fibre
Enhancing		**Active substance**
Liver/meat/fish	+++	"Meat factor"
Orange, pear, apple	+++	Vitamin C
Plum, banana	++	Vitamin C
Cauliflower	++	Vitamin C
Lettuce, tomato, green pepper, cucumber	+	Vitamin C
Carrot, potato, beetroot, pumpkin, broccoli, tomato, cabbage	++/+	Citric, malic and tartaric acids
Kefir, sauerkraut	++	Acids

Source: adapted from British Nutrition Foundation *(9)*.

heat treatment is thought to reduce the phytate content of tubers though not of cereals and legumes. Soaking and germination promote enzymatic hydrolysis of phytate in grains and legumes *(11)*.

The strongest inhibitors of iron absorption are phytates and polyphenols. Phytates are storage forms of phosphates and minerals present in cereal grains, vegetables, seeds and nuts. They strongly inhibit iron absorption in a dose-dependent manner, and even small amounts can inhibit the absorption of iron. There are a number of traditional food preparation practices that reduce the levels of phytates present in plant foods. These include fermentation, germination, milling, soaking and roasting. Phytates can be almost completely degraded by fermentation, which thus improves iron absorption.

Phenolic compounds exist in almost all plants as part of their defence system against insects and animals. A few phenolic compounds specifically bind iron and therefore inhibit its absorption. These are found in tea, coffee and cocoa, and also in many vegetables and several herbs and spices. The polyphenol tannin, which is found in tea, is responsible for the inhibitory effect of tea on iron absorption. Tea has been found to reduce iron absorption from a meal by 62% compared with water *(12)*. Indeed, tea has even been used therapeutically to treat iron overload *(13)*. In many European countries, and especially in the central Asian republics, it is common to introduce tea very early into the infant's diet. For example, a survey of children aged 0–3 years in Kazakhstan, Kyrgyzstan and Uzbekistan found that 21%, 34% and 49%, respectively, received tea *(14)*. Similar customs are found in central and western Europe *(15)*, especially among ethnic minorities. This practice will contribute to the development of iron deficiency.

Other factors

Iron stores are primarily regulated through changes in iron absorption. Injury to the intestinal mucosa due to the too-early introduction of unmodified cow's milk and dairy products can result in malabsorption, including decreased absorption of iron (see page 109) *(16)*. This can be pronounced in coeliac disease, which if untreated is often accompanied by iron deficiency anaemia. Chronic diarrhoeal disease is also a common cause of iron deficiency due to malabsorption. During systemic infections there is an acute decrease in iron absorption, paralleling a shift in iron from the circulation to the liver. This is a natural protective mechanism of the body during periods of infection, aimed at reducing the growth of harmful bacteria that require iron to proliferate.

Iron stores

Iron stores have an important buffer function in iron metabolism. At birth, iron stores are large and are gradually depleted over the first 6 months of life, after which maintenance of the infant's iron stores is dependent on dietary iron intake. The size of the iron stores can be assessed by measuring serum ferritin.

If the mother has severe iron deficiency anaemia, iron stores at birth will be small *(17)*, while moderate iron deficiency in the mother does not seem to influence the iron status of the infant. The size of the iron stores of the newborn infant are also influenced by the amount of blood transferred from the placenta to the infant at delivery, before ligation of the umbilical cord. Several studies have demonstrated a relationship between maternal anaemia and the risk of preterm delivery or low birth weight. Furthermore, preterm or low-birth-weight infants are born with the same ratio of total body iron to body weight, but because their body weight is low the amount of stored iron is also low. Moreover, preterm infants have an increased need for iron because of their need for catch-up growth after delivery. Preterm infants therefore need a good dietary source of iron earlier than term infants.

Growth
In the infant and young child, most of the absorbed iron is used for expansion of the haemoglobin, myoglobin and enzyme pools as the child grows. A 12-month-old infant is estimated to require around 0.3 mg/day of iron for growth (see Fig. 14). Rapid weight gain is therefore likely to be one possible cause of iron deficiency, and in some studies of healthy term infants rapid weight gain has been associated with low serum ferritin levels (5).

Iron losses
There is a small but continuous loss of iron from the body. This is mainly due to the turnover and loss of cells from the gastrointestinal mucosa and the skin (Fig. 14). Bleeding caused by gastrointestinal parasites, infections or the intake of unmodified cow's milk and other milk products before 9 months of age results in a loss of iron through the loss of blood. Feeding of unmodified cow's milk and other milk products during the first 6 months can cause bleeding of the gastrointestinal mucosa; furthermore, cow's milk has a lower iron content and bioavailability than breast-milk. The early introduction of cow's milk is thought to be the most important nutritional risk factor for low iron stores or iron deficiency in infants. This problem is most serious during the first months of life.

Hookworm infestation is a common cause of iron deficiency anaemia in many countries, and can be avoided through preventive measures and treatment (see page 121). Other infections causing blood loss are schistosomiasis of the urinary tract (*Schistosoma haematobium*) and dysentery. Many infections, especially malaria and chronic inflammation syndromes, cause anaemia but blood and thus iron is not lost from the body. Instead, as mentioned above, excess iron circulating in blood is transferred to the liver and stored there until the infection has subsided.

Physiological requirements and RNI
Age, gender and physiological status determine iron requirements. Iron required before 6 months of age should be provided by the iron stores of the infant and by breast-milk. After this, iron requirements must be provided by iron present in food. Requirements are especially high in infants from

the age of 6 months, in young children, and in pregnant and menstruating women. Blood losses during menstruation largely determine the iron requirements of non-pregnant women. The increased iron requirements of infants and pregnant women are needed to support growth and new tissue formation. A small amount of dietary iron (approximately 0.2 mg/day in a 1-year-old infant) is also needed to replace gastrointestinal and dermal losses *(18)*.

The physiological requirement (Table 31) for absorbed iron by young children is small compared with the amount usually present in the diet or compared with RNIs (Table 32). This difference is due to the low bioavailability of iron and the small percentage of iron that is normally absorbed: usually only 5%–15% of the iron in the diet. Absorption is influenced by the physiological factors described above and by dietary

Table 31. Physiological requirements for iron

Age/physiological status	µg/kg body weight/day	mg/day
4–12 months	120	0.96
13–24 months	56	0.61
2–5 years	44	0.70
Pregnant women	24	1.31
Menstruating women	43	2.38

Source: Verster *(19)*.

Table 32. Recommended nutrient intakes for iron in mg/day

Age	United Kingdom	United States	European Union[a]	WHO[b]
0–3 months	1.7	6.0	–	–
4–6 months	4.3	6.0	–	–
7–9 months	7.8	10.0	6.0	8.5
10–12 months	7.8	10.0	6.0	8.5
1–3 years	6.9	10.0	4.0	5.0
4–6 years	6.1	10.0	4.0	5.5

[a] Bioavailability 15%.
[b] Median basal requirement on intermediate bioavailability diet.

Source: Garrow et al. *(20)*.

factors such as the kind of iron (haem or non-haem) and the presence of enhancing and inhibitory factors in the diet.

The RNIs for iron given in Table 32 illustrate the large variations (from 6 to 10 mg/day at 7–9 months and from 4 to 10 mg/day at 1–3 years of age) that exist between the recommendations from different countries. These variations can be partly explained by the different eating traditions of different cultures and thereby differences in the sources of iron and its bioavailability, but they also highlight the scientific uncertainty regarding the optimal intake of iron for infants and young children.

Excess intake

A high iron intake may lead to iron overload, which is associated with a number of adverse effects. The absorption of non-haem iron is reduced, however, if the iron stores are high, and in most cases this is likely to protect the individual from iron overload. A normal diet can result in iron overload if the person suffers from hereditary haemochromatosis, which is characterized by lifelong excess absorption of iron from the diet. Among people of European extraction, hereditary haemochromatosis is the most common genetic disorder of excess iron absorption, with a prevalence of 2–5 per 1000 in the Caucasian population. For these people iron can be toxic, leading to tissue and organ damage and ultimately death.

Iron is a pro-oxidant, and increased consumption can potentially induce increased oxidative stress (21). This may explain why some epidemiological studies of adults have linked high iron stores, measured by high serum ferritin values, to an increased risk of cardiovascular disease (22,23), non-insulin-dependent diabetes (24,25) and cancer (26,27). The relevance of these findings to infants and young children is not known, and there are no studies in this age group linking a high iron intake with increased oxidative stress and adverse symptoms.

Several studies have shown an association between iron treatment and an increased risk of infection. As discussed above, the body withholds iron from microorganisms as a defence against infection. During infections, iron is displaced from the vascular bed to the liver and iron absorption is decreased. Iron administration during infections could thus increase the risk of infection. In most of the studies, however, iron was given parenterally, bypassing the regulatory mechanism of absorption. With the exception of malnourished individuals with infections, there is no convincing evidence that the oral administration of iron, either in the form of iron-fortified foods or as medicinal iron supplements, increases the risk or severity of infection *(8)*. In nutritional rehabilitation of severely malnour-ished children it is recommended not to start iron supplementation until one week after the start of treatment *(28)*.

High intakes of iron may interfere with the absorption of copper and zinc, since the three minerals have the same mechanism for absorption. Copper is likely to be most affected *(8)*.

In conclusion, a high iron intake can theoretically cause adverse effects, but there is limited evidence in infants and young children that a physiological amount of oral iron has adverse effects. In populations with a documented high prevalence of iron deficiency, the possible negative effects of giving excessive amounts of iron are outweighed by the well documented positive effects of preventing the symptoms of iron deficiency. In populations where iron deficiency is uncommon or where the iron status of the population is unknown, however, it is prudent to avoid too high an iron intake.

SYMPTOMS AND CONSEQUENCES OF IRON DEFICIENCY

Symptoms of anaemia range from nonspecific conditions, such as fatigue, weakness, dizziness and sensitivity to cold, to the clinical manifestations of chronic anaemia, which include changes to the fingernails, hair or tongue, breathlessness and heart failure.

The major consequences of iron deficiency anaemia include a higher risk of maternal mortality, fetal growth retardation, increased prenatal and peri-natal mortality, and lowered physical activity *(29)*. Atrophy of the villi of the small intestine, causing malabsorption, has been reported in iron-defi-cient infants. Appetite is reduced, which compounds the problem of im-proving iron status by dietary means, and is often accompanied by faltering growth and poor physical development in young children.

Iron deficiency has also been linked with increased susceptibility to infec-tion, although the relationship between the two is complex. There is good evidence that iron deficiency adversely affects cell-mediated immunity and causes a decrease in the bactericidal activity of neutrophils, thus lowering resistance and increasing morbidity.

In infants and children under 2 years of age, the consequence of iron defi-ciency of greatest concern is the possible impairment of mental and psycho-motor development. Infants are particularly vulnerable to iron deficiency during the period of complementary feeding (between 6 and 24 months of age) when the growth rate is high. This period represents the peak prevalence of iron deficiency in children, and coincides with the latter part of the spurt in brain growth when cognitive and motor development are taking place.

Evidence from community-based studies has demonstrated a positive association between iron deficiency and impaired performance in a range of mental and physical functions in children of different age groups, particularly infants. It has also been suggested that iron deficiency alters the emotional state of infants so that they are more withdrawn, cautious and hesitant, and as a result may be less able to interact and learn from their environment, thus hindering their intellectual development. In preschool children (36–72 months of age) iron deficiency has been associated with poor learning performance, particularly in tasks that demand close attention and discrimination of cues critical to solving visual problems.

The majority of studies of the effects of iron therapy in infants and children under 2 years of age report no improvement in the mental and physical development of anaemic infants after either short- or long-term administration, despite elimination of anaemia. In preschool children, however, iron deficiency has been successfully corrected with iron supplementation, and has resulted in a marked improvement such that the learning problems associated with anaemia disappeared. Thus the risk of permanent developmental deficits may be related to the child's age at the time of the deficiency or to the duration of iron deficiency (30), and the degree of iron deficiency is also likely to determine whether there is risk of permanent adverse effects.

To summarize, the evidence for a causal association between anaemia in infancy and poor neurodevelopment is not conclusive. Currently, only two intervention trials have been conducted. One failed to show that anaemic infants given prophylactic iron supplementation after 6 months had improved developmental scores compared with untreated controls (31). The second, carried out in infants who were more socioeconomically disadvantaged, did demonstrate such benefits (32). Iron deficiency anaemia is more common in conditions of biological (low birth weight, other nutritional deficiencies, high infection rates), psychological (lack of stimulation) or social (poverty, overcrowding) disadvantage (see Chapter 9). It is possible that the adverse effects of iron deficiency on mental development may be manifest only when infants are already vulnerable to other risk factors, and consequently the benefits of prevention are more likely to be observed in such children (2). Given the likelihood of long-lasting effects of iron deficiency during infancy, and the possible irreversibility of developmental delay through supplementation in some children, prevention is particularly vital and should be given a higher priority than detection and treatment.

COMPLEMENTARY FOODS AND CONTROL OF IRON DEFICIENCY

The bioavailability of iron is more important than the total amount of iron in the diet, and this should be taken into consideration when developing recommendations on how to feed young children. Examples of iron content and bioavailability in infant foods are given in Table 33. In the following section food items are discussed in the context of their bioavailability of iron.

Human milk

The iron content of human milk is low (Table 33) but it has a bioavailability of about 50%, which is much higher than that of other foods. The reason for the high absorption of iron from human milk is not fully understood, but it may be due to the lower phosphate and protein content of human milk compared to cow's milk and the high concentration of the iron-binding protein lactoferrin *(34)*. Owing to the iron stores present at birth and the high bioavailability of iron in human milk, exclusively breastfed full-term infants usually have a satisfactory iron status until about 6 months of age *(35,36)*.

Table 33. Iron content and bioavailablility in infant foods			
	Content (mg/100g)	Absorption (%)	Amount absorbed (µg/100g)
Cow's milk	0.02	10	2
Cooked rice	0.40	2	8
Carrots	0.5	4	20
Breast-milk	0.04	50	20
Fortified infant formula	0.6	20	120
Fortified wheat flour	1.65	20	330
Beef	1.2	23 (haem)	
	1.8	8 (non-haem)	460 (total)
Iron-fortified cereal	12.0	4	480

Sources: Hurrell & Jacob *(33)*; Lönnerdal *(34)*; R. Yip, personal communication, 1999.

Infant formula

If infants are not breastfed they should be fed a commercial iron-fortified infant formula. The level of fortification differs; in Europe it is typically 6–7 mg/l while in the United States it is 12 mg/l. More recent studies suggest that even smaller amounts of iron (2–4 mg/l) can prevent the development of iron deficiency in infants under 6 months of age *(37)*, but thereafter a higher iron content is needed. The iron compound in commercial infant formula, ferrous sulfate, is well absorbed (Table 33).

Cow's milk and other dairy products

In contrast to breast-milk, iron from unmodified cow's milk is poorly absorbed (Table 33). The poor bioavailability is likely to be due to the high content of protein and the low content of vitamin C compared to commercial infant formula. Furthermore, the early introduction of unmodified cow's milk and other milk products can cause blood loss from the intestinal tract, and thereby have a negative influence on iron status. Many studies have confirmed that cow's milk has a negative effect on iron status, especially during the first 6 months of life *(16,38,39)* and also during the last half of infancy *(5,16,40)*. A decrease (from 21% to 10%) in the percentage of Italian infants with iron deficiency was observed during a 10-year period when breastfeeding at 5 months increased from 22% to 51% and the consumption of cow's milk at 6 months decreased from 73% to 8% *(41)*. Similar observations have been made in the Russian Federation (O. Netrebenko, personal communication, 1997).

In this publication it is recommended that cow's milk should not be given as a drink before the age of 9 months. Thereafter, if infants are no longer breastfed, it can be introduced gradually. Infants who are neither being breastfed nor receiving a commercial iron-fortified infant formula should receive home-prepared cow's milk formula together with an iron supplement.

During the fermentation of milk, lactic acid and other organic acids are produced and these increase the absorption of iron. If fermented milk is consumed at mealtimes, these acids are likely to have a positive effect on the absorption of iron from other foods.

Other drinks

Fruit juices, if made from the flesh of fruit, have a high content of vitamin C, which has a positive effect on iron absorption if consumed with meals. Nevertheless, fruit juice in some countries does not contain vitamin C, especially if made by combining jam or fruit compotes with water. All the vitamin C is destroyed during the processing of jam and fruit compotes.

The consumption of tea, which is very common throughout many parts of the Region, has been associated with poor iron status because it has a negative effect on iron absorption.

Meat and fish

Meat and fish have a positive effect on iron status because they contain haem iron, which is highly bioavailable, and because they have a positive effect on the absorption of non-haem iron present in other foods in the same meal. Thus the available iron from a meal with vegetables can be improved considerably if a little meat is added. In one study of 7-month-old infants, the absorption of non-haem iron from vegetables was increased by 50% when meat was added to the meal *(42)*. Meat is not a major constituent of a complementary diet of most societies, and large amounts of meat introduced early will result in a high protein intake, which could have adverse effects. Only small amounts of meat are necessary to improve iron status, however, and meat should be introduced gradually into the diet from the age of about 6 months (see Chapter 8). In an intervention study of 8–10-month-old infants, a group receiving 27 g meat per day had significantly higher haemoglobin values after 2 months than those receiving only 10 g meat per day *(43)*. Meat is expensive, but because only small amounts are needed to improve a complementary diet economic constraints should not be a major limiting factor, especially if less expensive sources (notably liver) are recommended. If it is not economically possible to give meat daily, giving it only a few times or even once a week is beneficial. Liver, for example, is both cheap and high in micronutrients such as zinc and vitamins A, B and D, as well as iron. If puréed, liver therefore represents a good complementary food after about 6 months of age. Fish contains haem iron and therefore has a positive effect on iron status. Fish is also thought to contain a "meat factor" with a positive effect on non-haem iron absorption.

Cereals, pulses and vegetables

Non-haem iron is the principal form of dietary iron, and is found in foods of plant origin. The main sources are cereals, pulses, beans, vegetables and fruits. Cereals have a higher content of phytates than pulses and, as a result, pulses represent a better source of bioavailable iron. Iron present in leavened bread (made with yeast) has a greater bioavailability than that found in unleavened bread.

Iron-fortified infant foods

Iron can be defined as one of the "problem nutrients", for which there is a large discrepancy between the content in complementary foods and the amount required by the infant (44). The iron content of complementary foods, derived from family foods, is often low and has a poor bioavailability. Changes to complementary feeding practices, as recommended in this chapter and throughout the publication, will enhance the iron content of the diet and the bioavailability of iron in complementary foods, and thus improve the iron status of infants. Under some conditions, however, where there is evidence that the iron requirements of infants cannot be met by complementary foods derived from family foods, iron fortification of those foods will help combat iron deficiency.

Iron fortification of complementary foods for infants and young children is the most common form of targeted fortification. There is good evidence (45–47) that iron added to infant formulas and commercial baby foods is well absorbed and that fortified complementary foods can help to reduce the prevalence of iron deficiency in infants over 6 months and in young children (33).

Several different iron salts can be used to fortify foods, but there are differences in their efficacy in providing a source of absorbable iron and in their storage life. Although the soluble iron fortificants are readily absorbed, they tend to produce undesirable changes in the texture, flavour and smell of food. Ferrous fumarate and succinate have been recommended as iron fortificants for infant cereals because they are well absorbed and do not usually have these organoleptic effects. Milk-based foods may be fortified with ferrous sulfate. Sodium Fe-EDTA has also proven a safe fortificant for use in populations with endemic iron deficiency. It is stable, resistant to the common inhibitors of non-haem iron absorption and improves the absorption of intrinsic iron as well as zinc, but it is expensive (11). Moreover Fe-EDTA fortification should not be used in areas with a high level of lead contamination because of the risk of increasing lead absorption. Vitamin C can be added to counteract the inhibitory effect of phytate in high-extraction-rate cereal-based foods.

A promising approach is to use a multiple micronutrient formulation, especially when other nutrient deficiencies (such as that of vitamin A) are present. As yet, there is no agreement on what the composition of such a supplement should be, although it has been suggested that a powder could be added to complementary foods at household level.

OTHER INTERVENTIONS TO CONTROL IRON DEFICIENCY

A comprehensive programme to control iron deficiency and anaemia includes an appropriate mix of interventions designed to best address local
conditions, which are determined by the available infrastructures and depend
on the epidemiology of the iron deficiency anaemia. It is important to prioritize
programme efforts so that scarce resources can be used most effectively.

Reproductive and obstetric interventions

The iron stores of the newborn infant can be optimized by ensuring a
satisfactory iron status of the mother during pregnancy. Reducing the total
number of pregnancies and increasing the time between them has a positive
impact on the iron status of the mother. Because the iron cost of lactation is
generally less than that of regular menstruation, the promotion of exclusive
breastfeeding and thereby lactational amenorrhoea will contribute to the
control of iron deficiency anaemia in women of reproductive age *(48)*.

Scientific evidence also supports the view that the presence of maternal
anaemia does not prevent women from breastfeeding. Furthermore, lactation helps to reduce the likelihood of anaemia in a number of ways.

- Breastfeeding accelerates the contraction of the uterus to its size before
  pregnancy, thus reducing the risk of haemorrhage in the immediate
  postpartum period and thereby preserving maternal iron stores.

- The iron cost of lactation is generally less than that of menstruation, as a
  result of the lactational amenorrhoea produced by exclusive breastfeeding.

- The absorption of iron from the gastrointestinal tract is enhanced in
  lactating women.

- Lactation increases the mobilization of body iron stores in women.

If women are anaemic during the first half of pregnancy, the risks of low
birth weight, preterm delivery and perinatal mortality are increased *(18)*. In
addition, there is good evidence that severe iron deficiency anaemia during
pregnancy adversely affects the iron endowment of the infant at birth *(17)*.
A study from Jordan also found that maternal anaemia during late pregnancy was associated with a significantly higher incidence of anaemia in the
offspring *(49)*.

The high physiological requirements for iron during pregnancy are sometimes difficult to meet through the diet. There is therefore a general

recommendation that pregnant women should routinely receive iron supplements. The recommendations from the International Nutritional Anaemia Consultative Group (INACG), WHO and UNICEF are given in Table 34.

Table 34. Guidelines for iron supplementation in pregnant women		
Prevalence of anaemia	**Dose**	**Duration**
< 40%	60 mg iron and 400 µg folic acid daily	6 months in pregnancy
≥ 40%	60 mg iron and 400 µg folic acid daily	6 months in pregnancy and continuing to 3 months postpartum

Note: If 6 months' duration cannot be achieved in pregnancy, continue to supplement during the postpartum period for 6 months or increase the dose to 120 mg iron in pregnancy. Where iron supplements containing 400 µg folic acid are not available, an iron supplement with less folic acid may be used. Supplementation with less folic acid should be used only if supplements containing 400 µg are not available.

Source: Stoltzfus & Dreyfuss *(48)*.

Another low-cost intervention that can reduce anaemia in infants is the delayed clamping of the umbilical cord at birth. If the umbilical cord is not clamped and ligated until it stops pulsating (about one minute after delivery), more red blood cells are transferred from the placenta to the newly born infant. This process can help to prevent iron deficiency in later infancy, because it increases the body iron stores of the infant. According to a study carried out in Guatemala, infants with delayed cord clamping had significantly higher haematocrit values and haemoglobin concentrations at 2 months than those with early cord clamping *(50)*. Previous studies on delayed clamping expressed concerns that if the newborn was placed below the level of the placenta, adverse effects such as hyperbilirubinaemia, polycythaemia and diminished arousal might occur due to the excess transfer of blood. The study in Guatemala found no evidence of polycythaemia or other adverse health effects associated with delayed clamping when the newborn was placed at the same level as the placenta.

General fortification
General food fortification uses the existing food production and distribution system and, although this is not very costly, additional nutrition

education is required *(47)*. The following foods have been fortified: staple food (wheat flour), commercial infant formula, condiments such as sugar and salt, and milk and milk products.

The addition of iron to foods does not necessarily mean that it will be absorbed, or that it will help to prevent iron deficiency. Much iron added to cereal food today, particularly reduced elemental iron, is poorly absorbed. For example, soluble iron fortificants such as ferrous sulfate are absorbed to the same degree as the intrinsic non-haem iron in the diet. Iron fortificants are therefore poorly absorbed when added to cereal-based diets. Moreover, it should be remembered that the fortification of basic foods such as wheat flour also provides extra iron for adult men and post-menopausal women, who are often not iron-deficient; this could lead to an increased risk of atherosclerosis and cancer due to increased oxidative stress from the pro-oxidant properties of iron *(33)*. Furthermore, several studies have shown an association between high iron stores and cardiovascular disease and non-insulin-dependent diabetes mellitus.

Before introducing iron fortification programmes, the etiology of the iron deficiency in the target population must be established. Fortification of a foodstuff with iron is appropriate only if iron deficiency is related to low iron intake, low iron bioavailability or both and not, for example, to the presence of gut parasites *(29)*. While flour is a suitable vehicle for iron fortification in programmes aimed at older children and adults, infants and young children do not consume enough flour to achieve a significant positive effect on their iron status.

Supplementation

In some cases, supplementation with iron tablets or iron drops may be considered as one way to prevent iron deficiency anaemia, such as in children 6–24 months of age (see Table 35) and pregnant women, when given with appropriate dietary education programmes. Routine supplementation should be considered for high-risk groups such as preterm infants and infants receiving unmodified cow's milk and milk products before the age of 9 months. Major problems of iron supplementation are the lack of compliance in cases of long-term administration and gastrointestinal side effects, especially with higher dosages *(48)*.

Recently, several studies have compared the efficacy of weekly versus daily iron supplementation. Weekly supplementation resulted in limited side effects and limited risk of oxidative stress, and therefore represents a potentially useful long-term preventive measure as long as compliance is

Table 35. Guidelines for iron supplementation in children aged 6–24 months			
Prevalence of anaemia	Dosage	Birth weight	Duration
< 40%	12.5 mg iron and 50 µg folic acid daily	Normal	From 6 to 12 months of age
		Low	From 2 to 24 months of age
> 40%	12.5 mg iron and 50 µg folic acid daily	Normal	From 6 to 24 months of age
		Low	From 2 to 24 months of age

Note: If the prevalence of anaemia in children aged 6–24 months is not known, it should be assumed to be similar to the prevalence of anaemia in pregnant women in the same population. Iron dosage is based on 2 mg iron/kg body weight/day.

Source: Stoltzfus & Dreyfuss *(48)*.

good *(11)*. While research to evaluate these regimens in different population groups continues, the current recommendation remains daily supplementation for young children and pregnant women *(48)*.

Treatment of hookworm

In areas with endemic hookworm infestation, measures to control the parasite should be an integral part of iron deficiency control programmes. These might include prevention through better sanitation, screening programmes and mass treatment. The prevalence and intensity of hookworm infestation increase with age, so that its effect is greatest on the iron status of school-age children, adolescents and adults, including pregnant women *(48)*.

Screening for anaemia

Depending on its epidemiology, universal screening for anaemia is advisable in low-income areas, while selective screening should be used where the prevalence of iron deficiency anaemia is low. Because the iron stores of a full-term infant of normal or high birth weight can meet the body's iron requirement for up to 6 months, anaemia screening is of little value before this age. An exception is where unmodified cow's milk, which may provoke gastrointestinal bleeding, is used before the age of 6 months. In populations with a high prevalence of iron deficiency anaemia, however, monitoring and treatment programmes should be established.

The measurement of haemoglobin levels in primary care facilities should be reviewed to ensure that an accurate system with minimal reagent requirements is used. Strict attention must be paid to the use of sterile (preferably disposable) lancets for obtaining blood, owing to the danger of hepatitis and HIV transmission.

REFERENCES

1. DeMaeyer, E.M. et al. *Preventing and controlling iron deficiency anaemia through primary health care. A guide for health administrators and programme managers.* Geneva, World Health Organization, 1989.

2. Gillespie, S. *Major issues in the control of iron deficiency.* Ottawa, Micronutrient Initiative, 1998.

3. Department of Health, United Kingdom. *Dietary reference values for food energy and nutrients for the United Kingdom. Report of the Panel on Dietary Reference Values of the Committee on Medical Aspects of Food Policy.* London, H.M. Stationery Office, 1991 (Report on Health and Social Subjects, No. 41).

4. Siimes, M. A. et al. Exclusive breast-feeding for 9 months: risk of iron deficiency. *Journal of pediatrics*, **104**: 196–199 (1984).

5. Michaelsen, K.F. et al. A longitudinal study of iron status in healthy Danish infants: effects of early iron status, growth velocity and dietary factors. *Acta paediatrica*, **84**: 1035–1044 (1995).

6. Sherriff, A. et al. Haemoglobin and ferritin concentrations in children aged 12 and 18 months. ALSPAC Children in Focus Study Team. *Archives of disease in childhood*, **80**: 153–157 (1999).

7. International Vitamin A Consultative Group. *IVACG statement: vitamin A and iron interactions.* Washington, DC, Nutrition Foundation, 1996.

8. Fomon, S.J. Iron. *In*: Fomon, S.J. *Nutrition of normal infants.* St Louis, MO, Mosby, 1993.

9. British Nutrition Foundation. *Iron: nutritional and physiological significance. Report of the British Nutrition Foundation Task Force.* London, Chapman & Hall, 1995.

10. Hulthén, L.R. & Hallberg, H.L. Dietary factors influencing iron absorption – an overview. *In*: Hallberg, L. & Asp, N.G., ed. *Iron nutrition in health and disease.* London, John Libbey & Co., 1996.

11. Gibson, R.S. Technical approaches to combating iron deficiency. *European journal of clinical nutrition*, **51**: 25–27 (1997).

12. Hallberg, L. & Rossander, L. Effect of different drinks on the absorption of non-heme iron from composite meals. *Human nutrition: applied nutrition*, **36**: 116–123 (1982).

13. KALTWASSER, J.P. ET AL. Clinical trial on the effect of regular tea drinking on iron accumulation in genetic haemochromatosis. *Gut*, **43**: 699–704 (1998).

14. SHARMANOV, A. Anaemia in central Asia: demographic and health service experience. *Food and nutrition bulletin*, **19**: 307–317 (1998).

15. NORTH, K. ET AL. Types of drinks consumed by infants at 4 and 8 months of age: sociodemographic variations. *Journal of human nutrition and dietetics*, **13**: 71–82 (2000).

16. SULLIVAN, P.B. Cow's milk induced intestinal bleeding in infancy. *Archives of disease in childhood*, **68**: 240–245 (1993).

17. SINGLA, P.N. ET AL. Fetal iron status in maternal anaemia. *Acta paediatrica*, **85**: 1327–1330 (1996).

18. DALLMAN, P.R. Review of iron metabolism. *In*: Filer, L.J., ed. *Dietary iron: birth to two years*. New York, Raven Press, 1989, pp. 1–18.

19. VERSTER, A., ED. *Guidelines for the control of iron deficiency in countries of the Eastern Mediterranean, Middle East and North Africa*. Alexandria, WHO Regional Office for the Eastern Mediterranean, 1996 (document WHO-EM/NUT/177, E/G/11.96/1000).

20. GARROW, J.S. ET AL., ED. *Human nutrition and dietetics*, 10th ed. London, Churchill Livingstone, 1999.

21. SMITH, M. ET AL. Iron accumulation in Alzeimer Disease is a source of redox-generated free radicals. *Proceedings of the National Academy of Sciences of the United States of America*, **94**: 9866–9868 (1997).

22. SALONEN, J.T. ET AL. High stored iron levels are associated with excess risk of myocardial infarction in Western Finnish men. *Circulation*, **86**: 803–811 (1992).

23. TUOMAINEN, T.P. ET AL. Association between body iron stores and the risk of acute myocardial infarction in men. *Circulation*, **97**: 1461–1466 (1998).

24. SALONEN, J.T. ET AL. Relation between iron stores and non-insulin dependent diabetes in men: case-control study. *British medical journal*, **317**: 727–730 (1999).

25. TUOMAINEN, T.P. ET AL. Body iron stores are associated with serum insulin and blood glucose concentrations: population study in 1013 eastern Finnish men. *Diabetes care*, **20**: 426–428 (1997).

26. NELSON, R.L. ET AL. Body iron stores and risk of colonic neoplasia. *Journal of the National Cancer Institute*, **86**: 455–466 (1994).

27. STEVENS, R.G. ET AL. Body iron stores and the risk of cancer. *New England journal of medicine*, **319**: 1047–1052 (1988).

28. *Management of severe malnutrition: a manual for physicians and other senior health workers*. Geneva, World Health Organization, 1999.

29. GILLESPIE, S. & JOHNSTON, J.L. *Expert Consultation on Anemia Determinants and Interventions*. Ottawa, Micronutrient Initiative, 1998.

30. PARKS, Y.A. & WHARTON, B.A. Iron deficiency and the brain. *Acta paediatrica (Scandinavia supplement)*, **361**: 71–77 (1989).

31. LOZOFF, B. ET AL. *Does preventing iron deficiency anemia improve developmental test scores?* Ann Arbor, MI, Center for Human Growth and Development, University of Michigan, 1996.

32. MOFFATT, M.E. ET AL. Prevention of iron deficiency and psychomotor decline in high-risk infants through the use of iron-fortified infant formula: a randomized clinical trial. *Journal of pediatrics*, **125**: 527–534 (1994).

33. HURRELL, R.F. & JACOB, S. Role of the food industry in iron nutrition: iron intake from industrial food products. *In*: Hallberg, L. & Asp, N.G., ed. *Iron nutrition in health and disease*. London, John Libbey & Co., 1996.

34. LÖNNERDAL, B. Breastfeeding and formulas: the role of lactoferrin. *In*: Hallberg, L. & Asp, N.G., ed. *Iron nutrition in health and disease*. London, John Libbey & Co., 1996.

35. PISACANE, A. ET AL. Iron status in breast-fed infants. *Journal of pediatrics*, **127**: 429–431 (1995).

36. DEWEY, K.G. ET AL. Effects of age of introduction of complementary foods on iron status of breast-fed infants in Honduras. *American journal of clinical nutrition*, **67**: 878–884 (1998).

37. HERNELL, O. & LÖNNERDAL, B. Iron requirements and prevalence of iron deficiency in term infants during the first six months of life. *In*: Hallberg, L. & Asp, N.G., ed. *Iron nutrition in health and disease*. London, John Libbey & Co., 1996.

38. ZIEGLER, E.E. ET AL. Cow milk feeding in infancy: further observations on blood loss from the gastrointestinal tract. *Journal of pediatrics*, **116**: 11–18 (1990).

39. ROBSON, W.L. ET AL. The use of cow's milk in infancy. *Pediatrics*, **91**: 515–516 (1993).

40. ZLOTKIN, S.H. Another look at cow milk in the second six months of life. *Journal of pediatric gastroenterology and nutrition*, **16**: 1–3 (1993).

41. SALVIOLI, G.P. ET AL. Iron nutrition and iron stores changes in Italian infants in the last decade. *Annali del'Istituto Superiore di Sanità*, **31**: 445–459 (1995).

42. ENGELMANN, M.D. ET AL. The influence of meat on non-haem iron absorption in infants. *Paediatric research*, **43**: 768–773 (1998).

43. ENGELMANN, M.D. ET AL. Meat intake and iron status in late infancy: an intervention study. *Journal of pediatric gastroenterology and nutrition*, **26**: 26–33 (1998).

44. *Complementary feeding of young children in developing countries: a review of current scientific knowledge.* Geneva, World Health Organization, 1998 (document WHO/NUT/98.1).

45. RUSH, D. ET AL. The national WIC evaluation: evaluation of the special supplemental food program for women, infants and children. Background and Introduction. *American journal of clinical nutrition*, **48** (Suppl. 2): 389–393 (1998).

46. WALTER, T. ET AL. Prevention of iron-deficiency anaemia: comparison of high- and low-iron formulas in term healthy infants after six months of life. *Journal of pediatrics*, **132**: 635–640 (1998).

47. YIP, R. The challenge of improving iron nutrition: limitations and potentials of major intervention approaches. *European journal of clinical nutrition*, **51**: 16–24 (1997).

48. STOLTZFUS, R.J. & DREYFUSS, M.L. *Guidelines for the use of iron supplements to prevent and treat iron deficiency anemia.* Washington, DC, International Nutritional Anemia Consultative Group, 1998.

49. KILBRIDE, J. ET AL. Anaemia during pregnancy as a risk factor for iron-deficiency anaemia in infancy: a case-control study in Jordan. *International journal of epidemiology*, **28**: 461–468 (1999).

50. GRAJEDA, R. ET AL. Delayed clamping of the umbilical cord improves haematological status of Guatemalan infants at 2 months of age. *American journal of clinical nutrition*, **65**: 425–431 (1997).

Breastfeeding and alternatives

All infants should be exclusively breastfed from birth to about 6 months of age, and at least for the first 4 months of life.

Breastfeeding should preferably continue beyond the first year of life, and in populations with high rates of infection continued breastfeeding throughout the second year and longer is likely to benefit the infant.

Each country should support, protect and promote breastfeeding by achieving the four targets outlined in the Innocenti Declaration: appointment of an appropriate national breastfeeding coordinator; universal practice of the Baby Friendly Hospital Initiative; implementation of the International Code of Marketing of Breast-milk Substitutes and subsequent relevant resolutions of the World Health Assembly; and legislation to protect the breastfeeding rights of working women.

THE IMPORTANCE OF BREASTFEEDING

Human milk is the best food for babies and provides all the nutrients needed for about the first 6 months (26 weeks) of life. Moreover, it contains nutrients that serve the unique needs of the human infant, such as certain essential polyunsaturated fatty acids, certain milk proteins, and iron in a readily absorbable form. Human milk also contains immunological and bioactive substances, absent from commercial infant formulas, which confer protection from bacterial and viral infections and may aid gut adaptation and development of the newborn.

To clarify, "6 months" means the end of the first 6 months of life, that is when the infant is 26 weeks old, as opposed to the start of the sixth month of life (21–22 weeks of age). Likewise, "4 months" refers to the end and not to the start of the fourth month of life. Breastfeeding refers to breast-milk taken directly from the breast and should be distinguished from breast-milk feeding.

NUTRITIONAL BENEFITS OF BREASTFEEDING

Human milk is reliably superior to all substitutes, including commercial infant formula. The composition of human milk is not constant but changes during feeds, according to the time of day, and during the course of lactation. The total volume of maternal milk production and infant milk intake is highly variable, and although a mean milk intake by infants is often quoted as 650–850 ml per day, values may range from very little to more than 1 litre per day, depending almost entirely on the frequency and effectiveness of suckling. Breast-milk intake by the infant increases during the period of exclusive breastfeeding, reaching a plateau of about 700–800 ml per day after about 1–2 months, and only increasing slightly thereafter. The composition of human milk compared to that of commercial infant formula, cow's milk and home-prepared formula is shown in Table 36.

Table 36. Composition (per 100 ml) of mature human milk and cow's milk, and compositional guidelines for infant formula

Component	Mean values for mature human milk	Infant formula[a]	Cow's milk	Home-prepared formula[b]
Energy (kJ)	280	250–315	276	221
(kcal)	67	60–75	66	63
Protein (g)	1.3[c]	1.2–1.95	3.2	2.1
Fat (g)	4.2	2.1–4.2	3.9	2.5
Carbohydrate (g)	7	4.6–9.1	4.6	8.0
Sodium (mg)	15	13–39	55	36
Chloride (mg)	43	32.5–81	97	63
Calcium (mg)	35	59	120	75
Phosphorus (mg)	15	16.3–58.5	92	60
Iron (µg)	76[d]	325–975[e]	60	39
Vitamin A (µg)	60	39–117	35	23
Vitamin C (mg)	3.8	5.2	1.8	1.2
Vitamin D (µg)	0.01	0.65–1.63	0.08	0.05

[a] Acceptable range (one value only indicates minimum permissible values).

[b] Calculated assuming the recipe for home-prepared formula given on page 158.

[c] True protein = 0.85 g per 100 ml (excluding non-protein nitrogen), although a proportion of the non-protein nitrogen is used for the maintenance and growth of infants.

[d] Iron in breast-milk is highly bioavailable, with absorption of 50–70%.

[e] Iron in infant formula is poorly bioavailable, with only about 10% absorption.

Source: Department of Health, United Kingdom *(1)*.

Fat

Breast-milk has an energy density of approximately 280 kJ (67 kcal)/100 ml. Fat represents around 50% of its total energy content. The foremilk, at the beginning of each feed, is more watery and higher in lactose and has a relatively low fat concentration, which rises so that the most energy-dense milk is secreted at the end of the feed. This hindmilk therefore makes a vital contribution to the infant's energy intake. The fat-rich milk flows more slowly but provides important energy and nutrients, so feeds should not be ended when the flow of milk slows or the infant's suckling becomes less vigorous.

The proportions of fatty acids in cow's milk and human milk are very different (Table 36). Compared with cow's milk, human milk has a greater proportion of unsaturated fatty acids and a higher concentration of essential fatty acids. Furthermore, the long-chain polyunsaturated fatty acids (LCPUFAs) in breast-milk are better absorbed than those in cow's milk. Moreover, evidence suggests that LCPUFAs are important for normal neurodevelopment and visual cortical function. Because the newborn's capacity to convert essential fatty acids to LCPUFAs is limited during the first few months of life, infants rely on the efficient transfer of LCPUFAs from the mother, prenatally via the placenta and postnatally from breast-milk. Milk fats are also the vehicle for the uptake of the fat-soluble vitamins A, D, E and K (see below).

Carbohydrates

The main carbohydrate in human milk is lactose, which accounts for about 40% of its total energy, and is efficiently (> 90%) digested and absorbed in the small intestine under the influence of lactase from the epithelium. Unabsorbed lactose passes to the large bowel where it is fermented by colonic bacteria to short-chain fatty acids and lactate. These are absorbed and make a contribution to energy intake and reduce colonic pH, enhancing the absorption of calcium. In addition, lactose promotes the growth of lactobacilli and may help to develop a favourable colonic flora that protects against gastroenteritis. During acute gastrointestinal infection, formula-fed infants sometimes become lactose-intolerant due to epithelial damage and loss of lactase activity and may have to change to a lactose-free formula. Breastfed infants, however, remain able to tolerate the high lactose content of human milk and should continue to be breastfed *(2)*.

Human milk also contains significant concentrations of oligosaccharides. These components amount to around 15 g/l, and it is calculated that breastfed babies daily ingest several grams of oligosaccharides. Around 40%

are excreted in the faeces, and a small percentage (1–2%) in the urine. Since it is hypothesized that the remaining percentage is in part metabolized by the intestinal flora, there is speculation that these components act as a form of fibre in the diet of breastfed infants. These oligosaccharides may have a primary function in the defence against viruses and bacteria or their toxins and in promoting the growth of the colonic flora, including strains with possible probiotic effects such as the bifidobacteria.

Protein

The protein content of breast-milk is appropriate for the nutritional needs of infants. It is less than a third that of cow's milk. Moreover, human milk is whey-predominant, whereas cow's milk is casein-predominant with only 20% whey proteins. Of the human whey proteins, α-lactalbumin and lactoferrin are the most abundant, and represent a complete source of essential amino acids for the human infant. In contrast, the major whey protein found in cow's milk (and thereby in infant formula), is β-lactoglobulin, which is not present in human milk and can evoke an adverse antigenic reaction when fed to infants. The casein in human milk has chemical properties that make it easier for the human infant to digest than the casein found in the milk of other mammals. A proportion of milk protein, particularly in colostrum, is in the form of the immunoprotective proteins immunoglobin A, lactoferrin, lysozyme and other macromolecules that play a part in protecting the infant from microbiological infections.

Vitamins and minerals

Although women of marginal nutritional status can produce milk of adequate quantity and quality for normal infant growth, optimal micronutrient quality of human milk and therefore optimal micronutrient status of the infant depends on the mother having good nutritional status. To predict the risk of infant or maternal micronutrient deficiencies and the potential impact of maternal supplementation on breast-milk composition, and to plan appropriate interventions, it is useful to classify micronutrients in breast-milk into two groups (Table 37).

The concentration of those nutrients in human milk that are most affected by the mother's dietary intake are the water-soluble vitamins and, to a lesser extent, the fat-soluble vitamins. In contrast, with few exceptions, neither dietary maternal intake nor maternal stores affect the amount of minerals secreted in breast-milk. Where maternal intake can affect the secretion of nutrients into milk, there is usually a plateau above which a further increase in intake will have no effect in increasing their concentrations in milk.

Table 37. The effect of maternal intake and status on the micronutrient content of breast-milk

Micronutrients affected by maternal status	Micronutrients not affected by maternal status
Thiamin	Zinc
Riboflavin	Iron
Vitamin B_6	Folate
Vitamin B_{12}	Calcium
Vitamin D	
Vitamin A	
Iodine	
Selenium	

Characteristics	*Characteristics*
• Low maternal intake or status reduces the amount of these nutrients secreted in milk, and low breast-milk concentrations can adversely affect infant development.	• Maternal intake (including supplements) and deficiency have relatively little effect on their secretion in breast-milk.
• Infant stores of most of these nutrients are low and readily depleted, increasing the infant's dependence on a consistently adequate supply from breast-milk and/or complementary foods.	• Because milk concentrations are not reduced when the mother is deficient, she is vulnerable to further depletion during lactation.
• The concentration in breast-milk can be rapidly restored by increasing maternal intake.	• Maternal supplementation with these nutrients during lactation is more likely to benefit the mother than her infant.
	• Poor maternal intake or stores of these nutrients will have little effect on the amounts that infants will require from complementary foods.

Source: World Health Organization *(3)*.

Micronutrient deficiencies with clinical signs are rare in exclusively breastfed infants during the first 6 months of life. Provided that the mother's micronutrient status is satisfactory during pregnancy and lactation, exclusively breastfed infants under 6 months of age do not require vitamin or mineral supplementation. Where micronutrient deficiencies exist, however, dietary improvement or supplementation of the mother is likely to be effective, and will benefit both mother and infant.

Vitamin A

Vitamin A is vital for growth and for the development and differentiation of tissues, particularly the epithelia of the gastrointestinal and respiratory tracts. Human milk, and particularly colostrum, represents a good source of vitamin A. Breastfed infants rarely show signs of deficiency even at low intakes, but may have subclinical deficiency if maternal vitamin A status is poor.

Vitamin D

Vitamin D is primarily obtained through photosynthesis in the skin by the action of ultraviolet radiation. The vitamin D status of the newborn is dependent on the vitamin D status of the mother during both pregnancy and lactation. If it is poor, infant stores will be low and vitamin D levels in the breast-milk will be inadequate unless the infant receives sufficient exposure to ultraviolet light.

Folate

Breast-milk has a high folate concentration, which is maintained at the expense of maternal stores (4). Breast-milk folate concentrations do not fall unless the mother is severely depleted, and in the parts of Europe where supplementation of all pregnant and lactating women is a policy, folate deficiency is unlikely.

Iron

Despite the relatively low concentration of iron in human milk (which is nevertheless highly bioavailable) there is little risk of iron deficiency anaemia before 9 months of age in infants of normal birth weight who are breastfed exclusively for at least 4 months and who continue to be breastfed on demand (3). Iron concentrations in human milk are not correlated with maternal iron status and are relatively unaffected by the iron content of the maternal diet. Low haemoglobin levels or anaemia in the mother are not a contraindication to breastfeeding. In fact, maternal iron losses through milk during breastfeeding are less than those during menstruation. Thus, breastfeeding helps to prevent anaemia and anaemic mothers should be recommended to continue breastfeeding.

Zinc

Like that of iron, the concentration of zinc in breast-milk is relatively low, but it is highly bioavailable and is much better absorbed than zinc in commercial infant formula or cow's milk. The zinc requirement of formula-fed infants may thus be about one third greater than that of exclusively breastfed infants. Zinc deficiency is rare in exclusively breastfed infants before

6 months of age. During the first 6 months of lactation, the zinc concentration in human milk is unaffected by variations in dietary zinc intake (including supplements) or maternal zinc status in well nourished women. Consumption of non-breast-milk foods by an infant can significantly reduce the bioavailability of zinc and iron in breast-milk.

Iodine

There is little information on the iodine content of breast-milk in regions where dietary intakes of iodine are low. It is possible that in iodine deficiency the mammary gland sequesters enough iodine from maternal plasma to prevent breast-milk levels from falling significantly.

NON-NUTRITIONAL BENEFITS OF BREASTFEEDING

In addition to its nutritional benefits, breastfeeding also confers a number of non-nutritional advantages to young infants (Table 38). These include protection against various acute and chronic illnesses, and enhanced physiological and behavioural development. These effects have been evaluated in several reviews *(5,6,8)* and the most important are summarized below.

Infections

Breastfeeding protects infants from infections by two mechanisms. First, it lowers or eliminates exposure to bacterial pathogens transmitted by contaminated food and fluids. Second, human milk contains antimicrobial factors and other substances (Table 39) that strengthen the immature immune system and protect the digestive system of the newborn infant, thereby conferring protection against infections, particularly those of the gastrointestinal and respiratory tracts. Colostrum (milk produced in the first few days after birth) is especially rich in protective proteins, and should not be discarded.

The principal immunoproteins in human milk are secretory immunoglobulin A and lactoferrin. The former acts at mucosal surfaces to protect them from injury by ingested microbial antigens. The latter is an iron-binding protein that competes with bacteria for iron, reducing bacterial viability and thereby the risk of enteric infections, particularly those caused by *Escherichia coli* and *Staphylococus* spp. These immunological factors are not present in commercial infant formula or complementary foods. Formula-fed infants therefore enjoy less protection against infection. Human milk also contains many other defence and trophic factors that may play a role in the protection and maturation of the digestive tract.

Table 38. Health advantages of breastfeeding for infants and mothers

Infant
- Reduced incidence and duration of diarrhoeal illnesses.
- Protection against respiratory infection.
- Reduced occurrence of otitis media and recurrent otitis media.
- Possible protection against neonatal necrotizing enterocolitis, bacteraemia, meningitis, botulism and urinary tract infection.
- Possible reduced risk of auto-immune disease, such as diabetes mellitus type I and inflammatory bowel disease.
- Possible reduced risk of sudden infant death syndrome.
- Reduced risk of developing cow's milk allergy.
- Possible reduced risk of adiposity later in childhood.
- Improved visual acuity and psychomotor development, which may be caused by polyunsaturated fatty acids in the milk, particularly docosahexaenoic acid.
- Higher IQ scores, which may be the result of factors present in milk or to greater stimulation.
- Reduced malocclusion due to better jaw shape and development.

Mother
- Early initiation of breastfeeding after birth promotes maternal recovery from childbirth; accelerates uterine involution and reduces the risk of haemorrhaging, thereby reducing maternal mortality; and preserves maternal haemoglobin stores through reduced blood loss, leading to improved iron status.
- Prolonged period of postpartum infertility, leading to increased spacing between successive pregnancies if no contraceptives are used.
- Possible accelerated weight loss and return to prepregnancy body weight.
- Reduced risk of premenopausal breast cancer.
- Possible reduced risk of ovarian cancer.
- Possible improved bone mineralization and thereby decreased risk of postmenopausal hip fracture.

Source: adapted from Heinig & Dewey *(6,7)*.

There is abundant evidence that exclusive breastfeeding for around the first 6 months reduces both infant morbidity and mortality. These beneficial effects are more pronounced where infection rates are greatest and hygiene and sanitation are poor *(9–12)*, although benefits have also been found with respect to respiratory illness in industrialized countries *(13,14)*. In addition, infants tend to continue to accept breast-milk during episodes of diarrhoea, whereas consumption of non-breast-milk foods and fluids may

Table 39. Some protective and other bioactive factors present in human milk

Factor	Function
Secretory immunoglobulin A	Protects intestinal epithelium from luminal antigens, and may actively prime the neonate's immune system
Lactoferrin	Competes with bacteria for iron
Lysozyme	Antibacterial enzyme: lyses cell walls
Bifidus factor	Stimulates lactic acid bacteria, such as bifidobacteria, in the colon
Macrophages	Engulf bacteria
Lymphocytes	Secrete immunoglobulins (B cells) and lymphokines (T cells)
Protease inhibitors	Inhibit digestion of bioactive proteins in milk
Complement	Assists in bacterial lysis
Interferon	Antiviral agent
Oligosaccharides	Inhibitors of bacterial adhesion to epithelium
B_{12} and folate binding proteins	Compete with bacteria for these vitamins
Anti-staphylococcus factor	Lipid with anti-staphylococcal action
Anti-*Giardia* factor	Lipid with anti-*Giardia* action
Trophic factors	Accelerate gut development
Bile-salt-stimulated lipase	Improves fat digestion in the neonate
Docosahexaenoic and arachidonic acids	Constituents of cell membranes in brain and neural tissue
Antioxidants	Protect from free radical damage

decrease. Breastfeeding therefore both diminishes the negative impact of illness on nutritional status and provides a clean source of fluid to counter dehydration.

The concentrations of anti-infective substances in breast-milk are sustained beyond the first year of life and continue to offer significant protection against infection thereafter. In addition, the production of immunoproteins appears to be independent of women's nutritional and socioeconomic status (15). In a number of studies from countries with a high prevalence of infection, infants that breastfeed into their second year have significantly improved survival compared to those that have ceased breastfeeding (9,16–18).

The evidence that breastfeeding protects against infectious disease is greatest for diarrhoeal disease: formula-fed infants suffer a significantly higher number of diarrhoeal episodes than infants who are breastfed. The risk of necrotizing enterocolitis, a common gastrointestinal disease in neonatal intensive care units, is also greater in formula-fed infants than in infants receiving human milk, and the protective effects of breast-milk remain – at a reduced level – even when infants are only partially breastfed (19).

There is strong evidence that breastfeeding also protects against lower respiratory disease. In a recent study (20), breastfeeding was found to protect young children against pneumonia, especially in the first months of life. Formula-fed infants were 17 times more likely to be admitted to hospital for pneumonia than breastfed infants. Furthermore, a number of studies (21–24) have demonstrated a protective effect of breastfeeding against otitis media. Breastfeeding may also be protective against bacteraemia and meningitis (25–27), botulism (28) and urinary tract infection (29), although the evidence is less strong.

Active stimulation of the immune system

Most of the protective effects of breastfeeding against infectious disease are passive, that is, the immunoprotective factors in breast-milk protect the mucosal surfaces of the gastrointestinal and respiratory tracts and thereby reduce the risk of infection. There is also evidence, however, that breast-milk has an active influence on the infant's immune system. At 4 months of age, the thymus gland of breastfed infants is twice the size of that of formula-fed infants (30). Furthermore, the response to certain vaccines is better in breastfed than in formula-fed infants (31). There is also evidence that the protective effect against infection lasts for years after breastfeeding ceases. The factor in human milk responsible for the priming of the infant's own immune system is not known, but candidates are T and B lymphocytes, anti-ideotypic antibodies, cytokines or growth factors *(31)*.

Chronic disease
Studies investigating the impact of infant feeding on chronic illness are limited by their retrospective design. An inverse relationship between insulin-dependent diabetes mellitus (IDDM) and breastfeeding duration has been reported *(32–34)*. IDDM is an autoimmune disease, and it is possible that breastfeeding has a positive influence on the infant's immune system. Early exposure (< 4 months of age) to cow's milk protein may also act as a trigger for the early onset of IDDM *(35–37)*. There is also some evidence to suggest that breastfeeding may protect against Crohn's disease, ulcerative colitis *(38)* and childhood cancers *(39)*, such as leukaemia *(40)*. Further investigations are needed to confirm these claims.

Adiposity
It has been argued that breastfeeding prevents adiposity later in childhood. In a study from Germany *(41)* of more than 13 000 children, those that had been breastfed longest were significantly less likely to be obese at 5–6 years of age. Other studies have reported a similar effect.

Allergy
It has been hypothesized that breastfeeding protects against allergic disease *(42)*. First, human milk provides immunological factors that may protect the infant from exposure and reaction to antigens. Second, breastfeeding results in delayed exposure to many potentially allergenic substances present in foods. Breastfeeding protects against the development of cow's milk allergy, but the question of whether it protects against other allergic diseases, and whether protection against the symptoms of food allergy extends beyond the period of exclusive breastfeeding, remains unresolved *(43–45)*. More studies are required to define the complex relationship between infant feeding and atopic disease.

Sudden infant death syndrome
In several studies, lack of breastfeeding has been a significant risk factor for sudden infant death syndrome, and has remained significant after controlling for potentially confounding factors *(46,47)*.

Breastfeeding and cognitive development
Beneficial long-term effects of breastfeeding on IQ and cognitive development have been reported in several studies. In a meta-analysis of 20 studies comparing differences in cognitive development between breastfed and

formula-fed infants, breastfed infants had a three-point advantage after adjusting for confounders such as socioeconomic status and maternal education (48).

Maternal–infant bonding and infant development

Breastfeeding favours early bonding between mother and infant, and this is likely to play a key role in the development of optimal parental caring behaviour (49). Breastfeeding mothers may be more closely attuned and responsive to their infants than those who bottle-feed. Furthermore, it is possible that a young woman at risk of abusing her child might establish a more favourable relationship if given early support for breastfeeding, and this area deserves exploration (50). Beneficial effects of breastfeeding on long-term development and IQ have been reported in both preterm and full-term infants, but it is very difficult to distinguish the effects of feeding from those of other factors, including the parenting skills, IQ and education of the parents. A child that is not breastfed may receive less attention from and stimulation by his or her mother. Mothers who have chosen not to breastfeed should be encouraged to interact with their babies to the same extent as those who have, so as to facilitate bonding and to stimulate the infant's language and psychosocial development.

Lactational amenorrhoea

Lactational amenorrhoea refers to the inhibitory effects of breastfeeding on ovulation during the postpartum period. The duration of postpartum infertility is extended by breastfeeding in proportion to the frequency and duration of infant suckling. Suckling increases the secretion of prolactin and inhibits that of gonadotrophin releasing hormone. The interaction between prolactin and gonadotrophin-releasing hormone prevents the resumption of the normal pre-ovulatory surge in luteinizing hormone, thereby suppressing ovulation.

Reducing maternal fertility extends the intervals between successive pregnancies and leads to a decrease in the number of births, if other forms of contraception are not used. Increasing the space between births so that infants are conceived 18–23 months after a previous live birth (51) is strongly associated with improved child health and survival and has a number of positive effects on maternal health (Table 38). The contraceptive effect of breastfeeding is estimated to be 98% for the first 6 months postpartum, in women who are amenorrhoeic and either fully or nearly fully breastfeeding on demand (52–54). Exclusive, on-demand breastfeeding therefore represents a valuable method of contraception where other methods are not readily available or acceptable. It should therefore be promoted not only for the direct advantages it confers to the infant in terms of nutrition and protection from disease, but also for the indirect effects it exerts on maternal fertility and consequently on child spacing, and the health and survival of future children (55).

Breastfeeding and maternal postpartum weight loss

Investigations of the relationship between lactation and maternal postpartum weight have produced conflicting results, largely because of limitations in the design of studies. Of those studies that defined breastfeeding as lasting more than 3 months, however, the majority reported a positive association between weight loss and the duration of lactation while the remaining two found no association (7). There would appear to be no reliable evidence to support fears that breastfeeding increases the risk of maternal obesity, and it is likely that breastfeeding helps mothers regain their pre-pregnancy weight. Gradual weight loss (up to 2 kg per month) during lactation is normal.

IMPORTANCE OF MATERNAL NUTRITION

Women of poor nutritional status can produce sufficient milk of adequate quantity and quality to support normal infant growth. Nevertheless, maternal nutrient stores will be depleted and this can be detrimental if the intervals between pregnancies are short and there is insufficient time for them to be replenished. Furthermore, there is evidence that the fat content of breast-milk may be compromised if maternal fat stores are low. To ensure an optimal quality and quantity of breast-milk without compromising the health of the mother, it is thus important to optimize maternal nutritional status throughout pregnancy and lactation.

The increases in the mother's tissue mass and metabolic activity associated with pregnancy lead to an increase in her energy requirements. It has been estimated that the average energy cost of pregnancy for women with a pre-pregnancy weight of approximately 60 kg is around 293 MJ (70 000 kcal) (56). This apparent extra energy requirement, however, is rarely matched by an equivalent need to increase food intake, and direct measurements of food intake during pregnancy usually show only a small increase in the third trimester and virtually no change before then. The increase in energy requirements may therefore be balanced by a combination of (a) a decrease in activity to offset the increased energy costs of movement, (b) various energy-saving metabolic adaptations such as a reduction in postprandial thermogenesis and a reduction in basal metabolic rate, and (c) hypertrophy of the gastrointestinal absorptive surface area. Women should try to achieve a healthy body weight and optimal nutritional status *before* becoming pregnant, and while pregnant should aim for a desirable increase in body weight.

The energy costs of lactation are much more than those of pregnancy. The major determinant of the extra energy needed during lactation is the energy content of the milk produced. Assuming a milk production of approximately 750 ml/day and a gross energy content of milk of about 2.8 kJ (0.67 kcal)/ml, approximately 2.1 MJ (500 kcal)/day are secreted in milk. Additional energy will also be required to cover the costs of synthesizing breast-milk. It is therefore estimated that the additional dietary energy needs of lactation are approximately 1.4–1.8 MJ (325–425 kcal) per day above pre-pregnancy levels while full, on-demand breastfeeding persists and the extra maternal energy stores laid down during pregnancy remain available.

Good maternal nutrition during pregnancy and lactation to meet increased energy costs is therefore highly desirable. Nevertheless, there is general international consensus, based on scientific evidence from developing countries where protein–energy deficiency and undernutrition are widespread, that even underweight and/or anaemic women can sustain adequate milk production for as long as is recommended. Indeed, results from the majority of studies suggest that, unless the mother is both extremely thin (body mass index < 18.5) and in sustained negative energy balance *(57)*, adverse effects of undernutrition on lactation are unlikely.

In many parts of the WHO European Region there is a strong belief, often perpetuated by health professionals, that loss of maternal weight and/or anaemia are contraindications to breastfeeding. Consequently some health professionals believe that a large number of women are not capable of breastfeeding, and have discouraged it and instead have promoted the use of commercial infant formula. Health professionals require education and training to provide them with the information they need to reassure mothers that neither weight loss nor being underweight or anaemic are reasons for not breastfeeding. It is nevertheless important that women receive advice on how to improve their nutritional status. All women of childbearing age must be made aware of the importance of consuming a balanced diet, including plenty of fresh fruit and vegetables (more than 400 g/day). The training module on "Healthy food and nutrition for women and their families" *(58)*, including the booklet for mothers *Healthy eating during pregnancy and breastfeeding*, are available from the Regional Office and provide a useful guide, as do the CINDI dietary guide and the WHO food pyramid *(59)*. It should be remembered that low rates of breastfeeding in most countries of the Region are not due to physiological barriers but to social and psychological ones. Thus, improvements in nutritional status and the prevention of anaemia will not alone automatically result in improved breastfeeding practices. Ways in which breastfeeding rates can be increased are discussed in more detail on pages 146–152.

Substantial expansion of the erythrocyte mass increases iron requirements in the second and third trimesters of pregnancy and iron deficiency anaemia of pregnancy may be common, especially where iron intake or absorption is low and/or iron requirements are increased. It is therefore important to inform women which foods are good sources of iron and to recommend those that contain both iron and its enhancers. Excessive consumption of foods rich in inhibitors of iron absorption at the same time as foods containing non-haem iron should also be discouraged. Current recommendations can be found in Chapter 6, which is devoted to a fuller discussion of the iron needs and metabolism of the infant.

PRACTICAL ASPECTS OF BREASTFEEDING

Establishing breastfeeding

Immediately after birth the healthy baby instinctively searches for food. In the first couple of hours of life outside the womb, the baby is alert, active and ready to feed, and ideally breastfeeding should begin within the first hour. To facilitate this process, the baby should remain in skin-to-skin contact with the mother from immediately after birth until the end of the first feed. Mothers should be encouraged and helped to have skin-to-skin contact with their babies as much as possible during the first days after delivery, and mother and baby should be accommodated together. The practices that help and hinder breastfeeding are outlined in Table 40.

Good positioning of the baby's body is a prerequisite for good attachment at the breast and thereby adequate milk production and intake. Most difficulties can be avoided if good attachment and positioning are achieved during the first few feeds. Fig. 15 illustrates the difference between a well attached and poorly attached baby at the breast. The WHO/UNICEF training course on breastfeeding counselling (61) and WHO's practical guide for health workers (62) provide valuable information on attachment and positioning, and on breastfeeding in general.

Breastfeeding on demand is the key to establishing and maintaining optimum lactation. As long as the baby is adequately positioned and attached at the breast, and the mother breastfeeds frequently (8–12 times in 24 hours),

Table 40. Practices that help and hinder breastfeeding

Practices that can hinder breastfeeding	Practices that can help breastfeeding
Separation of mother and baby	Skin-to-skin contact between mother and baby
Delaying the first feed	Breastfeeding soon after birth (within 1 hour)
Restricting the frequency of feeding	Frequent, on-demand (baby-led) feeding
Feeding to a strict timetable	Letting the baby come off the breast spontaneously
Taking the baby off the breast before the baby is finished	Good positioning and attachment of the baby at the breast
Giving other fluids before the first breastfeed	Exclusive breastfeeding
Giving supplementary feeds of artificial milk	Exclusive breastfeeding
Giving plain water, dextrose, glucose or sucrose water or "teas" between feeds	Exclusive breastfeeding
Saying anything that makes a mother doubt her ability to produce milk	Building a mother's confidence through kindness and encouragement
Giving free samples of commercial baby milks	
Isolating the mother from those who support breastfeeding	
Using nipple shields, bottle teats and pacifiers	Avoiding nipple shields, bottle teats and pacifiers
Using drugs during childbirth that sedate the baby	
Washing the nipples before or after every breastfeed	Avoiding creams and ointments on the nipples; avoiding soap on the breasts and not washing them too often before breastfeeding

Source: WHO Regional Office for Europe *(60)*.

Fig. 15. A baby well attached (left) and poorly attached (right) at the mother's breast

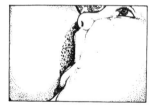 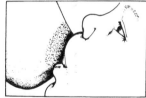

Source: World Health Organization *(61)*.

the infant is likely to consume an adequate amount of breast-milk. Babies have different feeding patterns and rigid feeding schedules are therefore not recommended. In hospital, truly unrestricted, on-demand feeding is only possible when the mother and baby are accommodated together, thus enabling the mother to respond when her infant shows readiness to feed.

Infants do not suckle continuously, and it is common for mothers to misinterpret pauses in suckling as a sign that the baby has stopped feeding, when in fact this means that the milk is flowing and feeding is going well. Baby-led feeding, in which the infant is allowed to spontaneously come off the breast when he or she is satisfied and chooses not to re-attach when offered the breast a few minutes later, will ensure the best milk production. Taking the infant off the breast prematurely, a custom in some places, can lessen milk intake, produce hungry babies, and needlessly lead mothers to doubt the adequacy of their milk production. Allowing the baby to drain the first breast before the second is offered will ensure that he or she receives optimal quantities of energy-rich hind milk. Breast-milk output is finely tuned to meet the demands of the infant, and a number of studies have demonstrated a positive correlation between breastfeeding frequency and milk output during partial lactation *(63)*. The frequency and completeness of milk removal are important local signals of the regulation of milk production, acting independently of systemic hormones such as prolactin. The build-up of a recently identified milk protein (feedback inhibitor of lactation hormone) is thought to inhibit milk secretion. Thus, frequent breastfeeding should stimulate milk production by limiting the accumulation of this inhibitory protein, whereas infrequent feeding allows its build-up in the circulation and thereby a reduction in milk output and possibly breast engorgement *(64)*.

Sustaining lactation

To sustain milk production, infants should suckle regularly and the intensity and duration of breastfeeding should be maintained. Colostrum, secreted during the first few days of life, is particularly rich in immunoprotective factors and some vitamins and minerals, and should not be discarded or withheld from infants in favour of prelacteal feeds. Exclusive breastfeeding provides milk of sufficient quantity and quality to meet the increasing needs of the growing infant until about 6 months of age. Even mothers of twins can exclusively breastfeed until around 6 months. When infant demand increases, and the mother responds by breastfeeding more often and longer at each feed, maternal milk production can increase within days and possibly within hours. Human lactation is flexible, and current evidence suggests that in most cases milk intake by a single infant is far below the mother's capacity for milk production. Practices that interfere with the infant's desire or ability to nurse effectively, such as the provision of supplementary fluids (water, glucose, dextrose or sugar water, teas, herbal drinks, juices, gripe water, milks and other fluids) are not necessary, will displace the richer, more nutrient-dense breast-milk, and will interfere with infant suckling and thereby compromise the establishment and continuation of breastfeeding. Even in warm climates, as long as they are exclusively breastfed, infants can conserve fluids and maintain adequate hydration without receiving any additional fluids.

In the first few months of life, irreversible milk insufficiency is rare. However, mothers often lack confidence in their ability to provide sufficient milk to meet their baby's needs and this fear is often reinforced by doctors and other health professionals. Anxiety may have a negative impact on milk secretion, and mothers thus need active and ongoing support to breastfeed well into the second year or beyond. Poor weight gain raises the possibility that the infant is not receiving enough milk from the mother. However, this may be an indication to improve counselling and breastfeeding support rather than to start using alternatives to breast-milk.

Methods of assessing the adequacy of infant growth are largely based on the use of "growth charts", and these should be used with caution. Some growth reference standards are outdated and are based predominantly on data from formula-fed American infants as opposed to international data from exclusively breastfed infants. Breastfed infants have different growth patterns (velocity) than their formula-fed counterparts (65), but there is no evidence to suggest the slower rates of infant growth achieved with exclusive breastfeeding for the first few months of life are suboptimal or harmful. Perceived poor nutritional status and "slow" growth, however, are reasons given for the premature termination of breastfeeding and inappropriate intro-duction of formula or transitional foods. New WHO standards based on exclusively and partially breastfed infants are currently being compiled (see Chapter 10).

Breastfeeding beyond 6 months

In the first year of life, the human body undergoes its most rapid phase of growth. Most healthy infants double their birth weight in the first 6 months and triple it in the first year, and at the same time body composition changes dramatically. Exclusive breastfeeding will fully satisfy the nutritional needs of most infants until about 6 months of age. As the baby gets older, bigger and more active, however, nutritional requirements can no longer be met by breast-milk alone *(3)* (see Fig. 1). Special transitional foods – comple-mentary foods specifically designed to meet the particular nutritional or physi-ological needs of the infant (see Chapter 8) – are needed to fill the gap between what is provided by breast-milk and the total nutritional needs of the infant.

The introduction of transitional foods does not mean the cessation of breastfeeding. On the contrary, for the first year of life breast-milk should continue to be a main source of food, and should preferably provide be-tween one third and one half of average total energy intake towards the end of the first year. The purpose of complementary foods is to provide *addi-tional* energy and nutrients, and they should ideally not displace breast-milk during the first 12 months. To ensure breast-milk volume is maintained, and to stimulate milk production, mothers should continue to breastfeed their infants frequently during the period of complementary feeding.

When expressed as an approximate percentage of total daily requirements, and assuming a range of intakes of breast-milk during the complementary feeding period, complementary foods need to provide 5–30% of vitamin A, 20–45% of protein, 50–80% of thiamin, 50–65% of riboflavin, 60% of calcium, 85% of zinc and almost 100% of iron needs *(3)*. The estimates suggest that almost no vitamin B_6, vitamin B_{12}, vitamin C or folate should be needed from complementary foods, because human milk has a sufficient content of these micronutrients. Human milk therefore represents a very valuable source of nutrients well beyond the time it ceases to be the sole provider of them.

There are a number of external factors that influence the length of time a mother is able to breastfeed her child. Of these, maternity leave and the breastfeeding rights of working women are of primary concern and have been highlighted in the Innocenti Declaration *(66;* and see Annex 1, page 272).

Women represent a significant proportion of the workforce in most European countries, and for many women economic constraints will mean that they must return to work while still breastfeeding. Return to the workplace forces mothers, and thereby infants, to conform to schedules that are likely to constrain the flexibility required for breastfeeding on demand. The frequency of breastfeeding is therefore likely to decrease, and consequently breast-milk volume can decline. Expression of milk (using hand expression or a pump) to be fed back to the baby and breastfeeding at night help to maintain milk production, and it should be possible to continue with at least two or three breastfeeds per day throughout the later part of infancy and beyond. The provision of crèche facilities and/or lactation rooms where mothers can express and store their milk, help mothers continue in their decision to breastfeed and will improve breastfeeding frequency. Furthermore, the establishment of crèche facilities in the workplace will benefit all mother–infant relationships, whether or not the infant is breastfed.

WHO and UNICEF currently recommend that breastfeeding should continue for up to 2 years and possibly longer. Evidence supporting the continuation of breastfeeding into the second year of life is strongest in settings where hygiene is poor and infection rates are high. In these conditions, prolonged breastfeeding (for up to 2 or 3 years) has been found to protect against infectious disease and to have a positive association with child survival *(16,17)*. In industrialized countries, the benefits of prolonged breastfeeding are less evident *(67)*. As a result, the American Academy of Pediatrics *(5)* recommends breastfeeding for at least 12 months and continuation as long as mother and infant desire, while European countries such as Denmark and the United Kingdom tend to give no recommendation on duration of breastfeeding beyond the first 6 months. For the WHO European Region it is therefore recommended that breastfeeding should preferably continue beyond the first year of life, and in populations with high rates of infection continued breastfeeding through the second year of life and longer will benefit the infant.

HOW TO INCREASE THE DURATION AND INCIDENCE OF BREASTFEEDING

Many factors affect how women feed their infants and the length of time they breastfeed them. These include traditional health care practices, the influence of family and friends, the living environment (urban or rural), socioeconomic status, maternal education, employment and workplace, commercial pressures, and knowledge and availability of breast-milk substitutes. Sociocultural factors also determine beliefs and attitudes, as well as practices, related to breastfeeding (see Chapter 9).

Women's perceptions of infant feeding are often formed before they become pregnant or give birth. They may vary with ethnicity, marital status and age *(68,69)* and prior experience, including how a woman was herself fed as a baby *(70)*. The baby's father and grandmothers are particularly powerful forces in influencing the mother's decision to breastfeed, and the pregnant woman's perception of her partner's attitude toward breastfeeding may also influence her decision. Around the time of childbirth, important influences include female peers – friends, sisters and other relatives *(71)* – and male partners *(72)*.

Breastfeeding rates are also influenced by cultural attitudes, which differ both between and within countries. These differences cannot be explained by socioeconomic factors alone. To improve the initiation and duration of breastfeeding it is essential to address local attitudes, but changing public perception of the best way to feed infants and young children is a big challenge. Health education programmes that promote the benefits of breastfeeding need to target both men and women at all levels of society, in order to bring about a change in the public's perception of the social acceptability of breastfeeding, in both private and public places, and cultural attitudes to it. Health education programmes in schools should stress the advantages of breastfeeding, and emphasize that the breast is an organ of infant nutrition.

Baby Friendly Hospital Initiative
Current health care practices are often at odds with recommendations on the best ways to successfully establish breastfeeding. The "ten steps to successful breastfeeding" shown in Box 3 are the foundation of the Baby Friendly Hospital Initiative launched worldwide by UNICEF and WHO in 1992 *(73)*. They summarize the maternity practices necessary to establish a supportive environment for women wishing to breastfeed and thereby to bring about improvements in the incidence and duration of breastfeeding. The Initiative also prohibits the supply of free and low-cost infant formula in hospitals, and demands the elimination of advertising and promotional activities for infant formula or bottle feeding. To become a baby friendly hospital, every facility that contributes to maternity services and to the care of newborn infants must implement the 10 steps.

Reinforcing this, the Forty-fifth World Health Assembly in 1992 urged Member States to encourage and support all public and private health

---

Box 3. Ten steps to successful breastfeeding

1. Have a written breastfeeding policy that is routinely communicated to all health care staff.

2. Train all health care staff in skills necessary to implement this policy.

3. Inform all pregnant women about the benefits and management of breastfeeding.

4. Help mothers initiate breastfeeding within a half hour of birth.

5. Show mothers how to breastfeed, and how to maintain lactation even if they should be separated from their infants.

6. Give newborn infants no food and drink other than breast-milk, unless *medically* indicated.

7. Practise rooming-in – allow mothers and infants to remain together 24 hours a day.

8. Encourage breastfeeding on demand.

9. Give no artificial teats or pacifiers (also called dummies or soothers) to breastfeeding infants.

10. Foster the establishment of breastfeeding support groups and refer mothers to them on discharge from the hospital or clinic.

---

facilities providing maternity services so that they become "baby-friendly". It should be recognized that mothers choosing not to breastfeed will also benefit from baby-friendly practices such as skin-to-skin contact, rooming-in and feeding on demand.

The effect of the Initiative on the duration of breastfeeding and the prevalence of infection has been examined in a large-scale study in Belarus (M.S. Kramer, personal communication, 1999). The majority of hospitals in the country were randomized to either implement the Initiative or to continue with traditional practice.

The training and continued education of hospital staff are central to the realization of the aims of the Baby Friendly Hospital Initiative. It is expected that all hospital staff and community workers will have a positive attitude to breastfeeding and be able to offer consistent and accurate advice in a language and style that parents understand. A woman's decision to breastfeed is significantly influenced by health professionals, and mothers should be given continued support, encouragement and advice on their decision to breastfeed, which could extend into the second year and beyond according to current WHO/UNICEF recommendations. There is strong evidence that conflicting advice from health professionals is related to early cessation of breastfeeding. To ensure consistency of information, local public health policies on child nutrition should be developed with the help of parents. In addition, governments are urged to implement the International Code of Marketing of Breast-milk Substitutes *(74)* and subsequent relevant World Health Assembly resolutions, and companies that manufacture breast-milk substitutes are urged to adhere to it (the full texts of the Code and of the relevant resolutions are given in Annex 1). Furthermore, health professionals should have good knowledge of the provisions of the Code because they have a number of responsibilities under it *(75)*.

The Code was adopted by the World Health Assembly in 1981 as a "minimum requirement" to be enacted "in its entirety" in "all countries". The Code does not try to stop the availability or sale of breast-milk substitutes, but it does seek to stop activities that persuade people to use them. Most importantly, it also protects children fed these products by ensuring that labelling is safe and that decisions are made on the basis of truly independent health advice. The key provisions are summarized in Box 4.

Since 1981, eight resolutions have been adopted by the World Health Assembly, further clarifying and strengthening the Code. Important provisions made in these resolutions stipulate that:

- follow-on milks are not necessary and complementary foods should not be promoted too early;
- obstacles to breastfeeding should be removed from health services, the workplace and the community;
- complementary feeding practices should be fostered from about 6 months of age, emphasizing continued breastfeeding and local foods;
- there should be no free or subsidized supplies of breast-milk substitutes in any part of the health care system;
- governments should ensure that financial support for professionals working in infant and young child health does not create conflicts of interest;
- governments should ensure truly independent monitoring of the Code and subsequent relevant resolutions; and

- the marketing of complementary foods should not undermine exclusive and sustained breastfeeding.

These resolutions have the same status as the Code itself and should be read together with it.

Box 4. Summary of World Health Assembly resolutions on the International Code of Marketing of Breast-milk Substitutes

1. No advertising of any breast-milk substitutes (any product marketed or represented to replace breast-milk) or feeding bottles or teats.

2. No free samples or free or low-cost supplies to mothers.

3. No promotion of products in or through health care facilities.

4. No contact between marketing personnel and mothers (mothercraft nurses or nutritionists paid by companies to advise or teach).

5. No gifts or personal samples to health workers or their families.

6. Product labels should be in an appropriate language and no words or pictures idealizing artificial feeding (pictures of infants or health claims) should be used.

7. Only scientific and factual information to be given to health workers.

8. Governments should ensure that objective and consistent information is provided on infant and young child feeding.

9. All information on artificial infant feeding, including labels, should clearly explain the benefits of breastfeeding and warn of the costs and hazards associated with artificial feeding.

10. Unsuitable products, such as sweetened condensed milk, should not be promoted for babies.

11. All products should be of a high quality and take account of the climatic and storage conditions of the country in which they are to be used.

12. Manufacturers and distributors should comply with the Code [and all the resolutions] independently of any government action to implement it.

Member countries of the European Union and countries joining the Union must harmonize their national legislation with that of the Union, including the European Commission's Directive on Infant Formulae and Follow-on Formulae *(76)*. Directives give instructions to countries on the transformation of their provisions into national law, but those instructions are not always absolute, leaving governments with some discretion. Compared with the Code, the European Directive has weaker labelling requirements. It applies only to infant formula and follow-on formula and not to breast-milk substitutes, bottles and teats, and it permits certain forms of promotion such as advertising in specialist baby care and scientific publications. There is therefore a fear in some accession countries that the adoption of the stricter Code legislation will prejudice future membership of the European Union. Although the European Directive contains mandatory language, however, it does permit member states to adopt more restrictive provisions in relation to advertising, and good examples exist in Denmark and Luxembourg.

Continued support for breastfeeding

Knowledge is only one of a number of factors that can influence a mother's intention to breastfeed, and it may not have much effect by itself. Giving information about the benefits of breastfeeding might influence those who have not already made a decision or who are undecided, but increasing social support may also be effective in enabling women to decide to breastfeed and to carry out their decision.

Continuing support to sustain breastfeeding can be provided in a variety of ways. Traditionally, in most societies, a woman's family and close community give her the help she needs – although practices in this respect are not always optimal. In many countries, however, young women lack positive role models from whom to learn breastfeeding skills. As societies change, in particular with urbanization, support from health workers or from friends who are also mothers, and from the child's father, becomes more important. Evidence suggests that full breastfeeding for the recommended time is consistently associated with support and approval from the male partner and the mother's mother *(77)*.

Both professional and peer group networks are therefore essential and should be developed to support, protect and promote breastfeeding. There is an urgent need to explore the potential of community groups and counsellors, since they may be more able than formal health services to provide the frequent one-to-one help that mothers need to build their confidence and to overcome difficulties. Throughout western Europe there are highly effective mother-to-mother support networks, some of which are now expanding into eastern Europe. Policy-makers should identify potential support systems in the community, such as churches and local nongovernmental organizations, and develop these as focal points for peer support groups. Furthermore, in order to attain the goals outlined in the Innocenti Declaration *(66)*, governments should develop national breastfeeding policies, including legislation to protect the breastfeeding rights of working women. This legislation should cover issues such as maternity leave and also ways to make women's working environments more conducive to breastfeeding, by for example the provision of crèche facilities and adequate nursing breaks.

CONTRAINDICATIONS TO BREASTFEEDING

There are few absolute contraindications to breastfeeding, although many have been cited in the past. The literature from the former Soviet Union includes renal failure, heart insufficiency, cancer, psychiatric illness, thyrotoxicosis, acute viral and bacterial infections, fever of unknown origin, and haemolytic disease of the newborn, but these are not now regarded as being contraindications. The principal contraindications are infection of the mother with certain viruses, especially HIV, and some drugs taken by women when they are breastfeeding.

HIV infection

It is now recognized that if an HIV-infected woman breastfeeds, there is a risk that her infant will be infected with HIV through her breast-milk. It is therefore crucial that policies are developed to reduce or eliminate this route of transmission.

In countries where commercial infant formula is available and affordable, and where sanitary conditions do not expose formula-fed infants to an excess risk of bacterial contamination, HIV-positive mothers are advised not to breastfeed. In many countries, however, and especially those with a high prevalence of HIV, this is not the case and there is an urgent need to develop policies to tackle the problem.

In September 1999, WHO, UNICEF and UNAIDS issued a joint policy statement on HIV and infant feeding (Annex 2), which takes into account the available scientific evidence of transmission through breast-milk and which promotes the fully informed choice of infant feeding methods by HIV-positive women. In 1998 these three agencies produced a set of guidelines *(78)* intended to help decision-makers define what action should be

taken in their own countries or local areas. Above all, health care professionals must ensure that the policies developed comply with human rights
agreements, and principally that:

> All men and women irrespective of their HIV status have the right to determine the
> course of their reproductive health, and to have access to information and services that
> allow them to protect their own and their family's health. When the welfare of chil-
> dren is concerned, decisions should be made that are in keeping with children's best
> interest.

The overall objective is to prevent HIV transmission through breast-milk
while continuing to protect, promote and support breastfeeding for HIV-
negative women and those of unknown HIV status. The issues are
multisectoral and will be of relevance to decision-makers in a number of
fields including health, nutrition, family planning, education and social
welfare. A fuller discussion of ways to prevent mother-to-child transmission of HIV, together with the key elements required to establish a policy
on HIV and infant feeding, can be found in Annex 2.

Environmental contamination

Concerns have been raised about the risks to infants from breast-milk
contaminated by environmental pollutants. However, the risks of continued exposure to a chemical through breastfeeding have to be balanced against the risks of infection or nutritional deprivation when
breastfeeding is curtailed or discontinued (79). Thus, despite the presence of polychlorinated biphenyls, dioxins and furans in human milk,
breastfeeding should be encouraged and promoted because of the
convincing evidence of the benefits of human milk to the overall health
and development of infants (80). Furthermore, no major studies have
demonstrated that pesticides at the concentrations found in breast-milk
lead to adverse health outcomes in children exposed through
breastfeeding (81).

Therapeutic drugs

Most therapeutic drugs given to a lactating mother are excreted in her milk.
While in general drugs should be avoided if not necessary, there are only a
few drugs for which it is necessary to stop or postpone breastfeeding.
Among these are anticancer drugs (antimetabolites) and radioactive substances (Table 41). Some drugs (such as ergotamine) may be toxic to the
infant, some (such as estrogens) inhibit lactation, while others (such as
phenobarbitone) inhibit suckling. Often it is possible to use an alternative
drug or to continue breastfeeding while observing the infant for possible

Table 41. Breastfeeding and maternal medication

Breastfeeding contraindicated	Anticancer drugs (antimetabolites) Radioactive substances (stop breastfeeding temporarily)
Continue breastfeeding	
Side effects possible Monitor baby for drowsiness	Psychiatric drugs and anticonvulsants
Use alternative drug if possible	Chloramphenicol, tetracyclines, metronidazole Quinolone antibiotics (e.g. ciprofloxacin)
Monitor baby for jaundice	Sulfonamides, dapsone Sulfamethoxazole + trimethoprim (cotrimoxazole) Sulfadoxine + pyrimethamine (Fansidar)
Use alternative drug	Estrogens, including estrogen-containing contraceptives Thiazide diuretics Ergometrine

Safe in usual dosage: monitor baby	Most commonly used drugs:
	Analgesics and antipyretics: short
	  courses of paracetamol, acetylsalicylic
	  acid, ibuprofen; occasional doses of
	  morphine and pethidine
	Antibiotics: ampicillin, amoxicillin,
	  cloxacillin and other penicillins
	Erythromycin
	Anti-tuberculars, anti-leprotics (see
	  dapsone above)
	Antimalarials (except mefloquine,
	  Fansidar), anthelminthics
	Antifungals
	Bronchodilators (e.g. salbutamol),
	  corticosteroids
	Antihistamines, antacids, drugs for
	  diabetes
	Most antihypertensives, digoxin
	Nutritional supplements of iodine, iron,
	  vitamins

Source: WHO/UNICEF *(82)*.

side effects. Furthermore, it is possible that drugs in breast-milk can cause hypersensitivity in the infant even when concentrations are too low to cause a pharmacological effect.

Illegal drug use
The avoidance of breastfeeding is recommended where mothers are using illegal drugs.

Tuberculosis
Women with tuberculosis who choose to breastfeed should receive a full course of chemotherapy. Timely and properly used chemotherapy is the best way to prevent transmission of tubercle bacilli to the baby. All anti-tuberculosis drugs are compatible with breastfeeding and a woman taking them can safely breastfeed her baby. The exception is in women with newly diagnosed active tuberculosis infection, who should be advised to discontinue breastfeeding until they have received at least 2 weeks of chemotherapy. The baby should receive isoniazid prophylaxis and BCG immunization *(83)*.

Hepatitis B and C
Breast-milk can contain hepatitis B surface antigen (HBsAg), and it has been suggested that breastfeeding represents a route by which infants may acquire hepatitis B virus infection. There is no evidence, however, that breastfeeding increases the risk of transmission to the infant *(84)*. Hepatitis B vaccine will substantially reduce perinatal transmission, and could eliminate risk of transmission through breastfeeding. Even when hepatitis C virus has been detected in breast-milk, breastfed infants have not been infected and mothers positive for hepatitis C virus RNA should be advised to breastfeed *(85,86)*.

Smoking
Nicotine can reduce the volume of human milk produced and inhibit its release, and may also cause irritability and poor weight gain in infancy. Women who smoke have lower circulating prolactin levels, which may shorten the period of lactation and reduce the duration of lactational amen-orrhoea. Also, the vitamin C concentration in the milk of smoking mothers tends to be lower than that in the milk of nonsmokers *(87)*. Breastfeeding mothers should be encouraged to stop or reduce smoking, but breastfeeding remains the best feeding choice even when smoking continues. Smoking after a breastfeed rather than before will reduce the level of harmful substances in breast-milk.

ALTERNATIVES TO BREASTFEEDING

Breastfeeding is normally the best way to feed infants. Nevertheless, there are situations where it may be preferable or necessary to substitute breast-milk with an alternative. In addition to the contraindications summarized above, there will be situations where the mother, despite efforts to continue breastfeeding, will not be able to maintain lactation that will fully meet the infant's nutritional requirements. When cessation of breastfeeding is considered, the risk of giving other than breast-milk should be less than the potential risks associated with continued breastfeeding. Before starting giving other than breast-milk, it is vital to consider the following issues.

- Feeding needs to provide all the infant's nutritional requirements as completely as possible. No substitute fully replicates the nutrient content of breast-milk.

- Breast-milk substitutes lack the properties of breast-milk that protect against infection. Bacteria may contaminate breast-milk substitutes during preparation, and it is essential that feeds are prepared and given hygienically (see Chapter 12). Even when hygiene is good, artificially fed infants suffer a significantly higher rate of gastrointestinal and respiratory infections than breastfed infants.

- The use of breast-milk substitutes is expensive. A recent study conducted in the United States (88) estimated the cost of using a breast-milk alternative to be approximately US $800 for the first year of life. This cost has to be borne by individual families and translates into costs to communities, with an impact at the population level. In addition to formula, the costs of fuel, water and health care need to be taken into account.

- Women who do not breastfeed lose the benefits of lactational amenorrhoea. In populations where contraceptives are not readily available, this will potentially translate into short birth intervals and compromised maternal health unless women have easy access to family planning services soon after delivery.

- Not breastfeeding can affect mother–infant bonding, resulting in lack of stimulation for the infant. Mothers should be helped to ensure that non-breastfed infants receive as much attention as breastfed infants.

Commercial infant formula

Most commercial infant formulas are based on cow's milk, and have been designed to mimic the nutrient composition of human milk. Thus the concentrations of protein and of electrolytes such as sodium, potassium and chloride are lower than those in cow's milk, while the levels of certain minerals, primarily iron and to a lesser extent zinc, are higher (Table 36). Commercial infant formulas lack the non-nutritional, bioactive components of human milk (protective and trophic factors), and the quality of their proteins and lipids (amino acid and fatty acid profiles) may not be optimal for the needs of the baby (see below). Nevertheless, commercial infant formulas provide a satisfactory alternative sole source of nutrition to young infants up to about 6 months of age. Even after the introduction of complementary foods, formula continues to make a major contribution to infant energy and nutrient requirements and, *in the absence of breastfeeding*, it should be the main fluid in the diet for the first 9 months and possibly beyond.

Commercial infant formula is usually available as a milk powder that has to be reconstituted with water. The instructions on the tin or carton for preparing the formula should be followed *exactly* to ensure that it is not too concentrated or diluted. Overconcentration can overload the infant with salts and protein, which can be dangerous, and overdilution can lead to malnutrition. Health workers should be able to demonstrate to mothers and families how to make up breast-milk substitutes properly.

Compositional guidelines for commercial infant formulas have been agreed in the Codex Alimentarius, and these are defined according to the energy density of feeds, that is the energy per 100 ml using products with 65 kcal/100 ml as typical. It must be stressed that when commercial infant formula is recommended as the best alternative to breastfeeding, it is assumed that the formula meets the standards dictated in the Codex *(89)*. In some countries, however, commercial infant formula may be substandard owing to the absence of, or lack of enforcement of, national regulations.

Cow's milk and milk from other animals

Cow's milk

Infants should not be given unmodified cow's milk *as a drink* before the age of 9 months. If infants are fed formula, cow's milk can be gradually introduced into their diet between the ages of 9 and 12 months. If there are no economic constraints, however, it may be better to continue with formula until 12 months of age.

Cow's milk differs greatly from human milk in both the quality and quantity of nutrients, and lacks the trophic and immunological factors present in human milk (Table 36). In terms of nutrients, whole cow's milk contains greater amounts of protein and minerals (calcium, sodium, phosphorus, chloride, magnesium and potassium) and less carbohydrate, essential fatty acids (linoleic and α-linolenic acids) and long-chain polyunsaturated fatty acids, iron, zinc, vitamin C and niacin. Not only does cow's milk have a higher concentration of total protein, but its quality differs from human milk and its proteins are potentially allergenic to the human infant.

Home-prepared formulas

Milk formulas prepared at home from cow's milk, or that of other mammals such as goats and sheep, are sometimes used to feed infants. These are often deficient in many nutrients, most importantly iron, which is present in low levels and has poor bioavailability. Home-prepared formulas may cause gastrointestinal bleeding if based on unmodified cow's milk (see Chapter 6). They should be given only when commercial infant formula is not available. Nevertheless, they offer a better alternative than unmodified cow's milk. The younger the infant, the more important it is that he or she receives infant formula as opposed to cow's milk. If there are economic constraints limiting the availability of commercial infant formula, the use of formula should be given priority in the first months after birth, because these are the most important from the point of view of optimal infant nutrition and development. Where commercial iron-fortified infant formula is not available, fresh animal milks or dried milk should be modified according to the recipes below, and iron supplements should be given. Preparations of other micronutrients (such as zinc, which may be sprinkled on foods) are currently being developed, and may in the future offer a way of improving the micronutrient density of home-prepared formulas.

Modified animal milks

Because cow's milk has a higher solute load than human milk, it must be diluted with boiled water to reduce its concentration. This will have a negative impact on energy density, and therefore sugar should be added.

WHO recommends the following recipe for home-prepared formula (60).

- Boil 70 ml of water.
- Add 130 ml of boiled cow's or goat's milk to make 200 ml of feed.
- Add 1 level teaspoonful (5 g) of sugar.

This recipe can also be used if the milk is made up from tinned whole milk powder. The milk should be prepared according to the instructions on the label and then modified following the recipe above.

Goat's milk should be modified in the same way as cow's milk. Sheep's milk, however, has a very high protein content and therefore requires more dilution. The following recipe should be used when modifying sheep's milk.

- Boil 100 ml of water.
- Add 100 ml of boiled sheep's milk to make 200 ml of feed.
- Add 1 level teaspoonful (5 g) of sugar.

Like cow's milk, both goat's and sheep's milk are low in iron and vitamin D, and are also low in folate compared with human and cow's milk. While goat's milk is comparatively low in vitamin A, sheep's milk contains more than cow's milk.

Unmodified goat's and sheep's milk should not be given to infants under the age of 1 year, and thereafter only if precautions against mineral and vitamin deficiencies have been taken, together with action to ensure micro-biological safety.

Unsuitable breast-milk substitutes
Skimmed and semi-skimmed milk are not recommended for feeding infants under the age of 1 year. Skimmed milk has had most of the fat removed, and semi-skimmed milk about half of the fat removed, and neither provides enough energy for the growing infant. Sweetened condensed milk is also not recommended owing to its high sugar content. Fruit juices, sugar-water and dilute cereal gruels are sometimes given instead of milk feeds, but these are not recommended as alternatives because of their nutritional incompleteness.

Bottles and cups
Bottles and artificial teats are one method of feeding infants when they cannot be fed directly from the breast. Cup feeding, however, is becoming increasingly popular and is particularly recommended in areas where hygiene is poor, and for feeding infants under special conditions.

Both bottles and artificial teats can be harmful because:

- bottle feeding increases the risk of diarrhoea (where hygiene is poor), dental disease and otitis media, and may change oral dynamics;
- bottle feeding increases the risk that the infant will receive inadequate stimulation and attention during feeds;
- bottles and teats need to be thoroughly cleaned with a brush and then boiled to sterilize them and this takes time and fuel;

- sweetened solids are often added to bottle feeds and this increases the risk of dental caries, as does the practice of dipping pacifiers and teats in honey or sugar; and
- bottles may cause "nipple confusion", which may compromise breastfeeding frequency and intensity.

An alternative method of feeding infants who cannot breastfeed is by cup. This is recommended particularly for infants who are expected to breastfeed later, and in situations where hygienic care of bottles and teats is difficult. The correct technique for cup feeding allows the infant to control intake; milk should not be "poured" into the mouth.

The arguments in favour of cup feeding are that:

- the risk of poor attachment to the breast is less;
- the baby uses his or her tongue while feeding;
- cup feeding is baby-led, the baby pacing his or her own intake in time and quantity;
- cups are safer than bottles because they are easier to clean with soap and water;
- cups are less likely than bottles to be carried around for a long time, thereby giving bacteria the opportunity to multiply;
- cup feeding requires the mother or other caregiver to hold and have more contact with the infant, thus providing more psychosocial stimulation than bottle feeding; and
- cup feeding is better than feeding with a cup and spoon, because spoon feeding takes longer and the mother may stop before the infant has had enough.

The way to feed an infant with a cup is as follows *(90)*.

- Hold the infant sitting upright or semi-upright on your lap.
- Support the infant's back and neck with one arm.
- Hold the small cup of milk to the infant's lips.
- Tip the cup so that the milk just reaches the infant's lips. The cup rests lightly on the infant's lower lip, and the edges of the cup touch the outer part of the infant's upper lip.
- The infant becomes alert and opens his or her mouth and eyes. A low-birth-weight infant will start to take the milk into his or her mouth with the tongue. A full-term or older infant sucks or sips the milk, spilling some of it.
- DO NOT POUR the milk into the infant's mouth. Just hold the cup to the infant's lips and let him or her take it.

- When infants have had enough, they will close their mouth and will not take any more. An infant who has not taken enough may take more the next time, or the frequency of feeding may need to be increased.
- Do not try to make the infant drink a certain amount. Let the infant decide when he or she has had enough.
- Measure the infant's intake over 24 hours rather than at each feeding.

Pacifiers

Pacifiers are used worldwide and are believed by some health professionals and lay people to be harmless or even necessary and beneficial for an infant's development *(91)*. However, as with artificial teats, pacifiers may reduce the time spent suckling at the breast and thereby interfere with demand feeding, resulting in suppression of breast-milk production. They may alter oral dynamics and affect language development. Furthermore, pacifiers are frequently infected with *Candida albicans* and some children who use pacifiers may have oral thrush, which may resist treatment until the pacifier is discarded. Moreover, pacifiers may affect care because they are used as substitutes by caregivers for time and attention. If used, pacifiers should not be dipped into sweet foods such as jams and honey because of the risk of dental caries (see Chapter 11).

REFERENCES

1. DEPARTMENT OF HEALTH, UNITED KINGDOM. *Weaning and the weaning diet. Report of the Working Group on the Weaning Diet of the Committee on Medical Aspects of Food Policy.* London, H.M. Stationery Office, 1994 (Report on Health and Social Subjects, No. 45).
2. LAWRENCE, P.B. Breast milk: best source of nutrition for term and preterm infants. *Pediatric clinics of North America,* **41**: 925–941 (1994).
3. *Complementary feeding of young children in developing countries: a review of current scientific knowledge.* Geneva, World Health Organization, 1998 (document WHO/NUT/98.1).
4. O'CONNOR, D.L. Folate status during pregnancy and lactation. *In*: Allen, L.H. et al., ed. *Nutrient regulation during pregnancy, lactation and infant growth.* New York, Plenum Press, 1994, pp. 157–172.
5. AMERICAN ACADEMY OF PEDIATRICS. Working Group on Breastfeeding. Breastfeeding and the use of human milk. *Pediatrics,* **100**: 1035–1039 (1997).
6. HEINIG, M.J. & DEWEY, K.G. Health advantages of breastfeeding for infants: a critical review. *Nutrition research reviews,* **9**: 89–110 (1996).
7. HEINIG, M.J. & DEWEY, K.G. Health effects of breastfeeding for mothers: a critical review. *Nutrition research reviews,* **10**: 35–56 (1997).

8. GOLDING, J. Breastfeeding: benefits and hazards. Methodology and summary of results. *Early human development,* **49** (Suppl.): S45–S74 (1997).
9. VICTORA, C.G. ET AL. Evidence for protecting by breast-feeding against infant deaths from infectious diseases in Brazil. *Lancet,* **2**: 319–322 (1987).
10. BRIEND, A. ET AL. Breastfeeding, nutritional state, and child survival in rural Bangladesh. *British medical journal,* **296**: 879–882 (1988).
11. FORSYTH, J.S. The relationship between breast-feeding and infant health and development. *Proceedings of the Nutrition Society,* **54**: 407–418(1995).
12. WILSON, A.C. ET AL. Relation of infant diet to childhood health: seven year follow up of cohort of children in Dundee infant feeding study. *British medical journal,* **346**: 21–25 (1998).
13. CUSHING, A.H. ET AL. Breastfeeding reduces the risk of respiratory illness in infants. *American journal of epidemiology,* **147**: 863–870 (1999).
14. HOWIE, P.W. ET AL. Protective effect of breastfeeding against infection. *British medical journal,* **300**: 11–16 (1990).
15. WEAVER, L.T. ET AL. Human milk IgA concentrations during the first year of lactation. *Archives of disease in childhood,* **78**: 235–239 (1998).
16. BRIEND, A. & BARI, A. Breastfeeding improves survival, but not nutritional status, of 12–35 month old children in rural Bangladesh. *European journal of clinical nutrition,* **43**: 603–608 (1989).
17. MØLBAK, K. ET AL. Prolonged breastfeeding, diarrhoeal disease, and survival of children in Guinea-Bissau. *British medical journal,* **308**:1403–1406 (1994).
18. MITRA, A.K. & RABBANI, F. The importance of breastfeeding in minimising mortality and morbidity from diarrhoeal diseases: the Bangladesh perspective. *Journal of diarrhoeal disease research,* **13**: 1–7 (1995).
19. SCHANLER, R.J. & ATKINSON, S.A. Effects of nutrients in human milk on the recipient premature infant. *Journal of mammary gland biology and neoplasia,* **4**: 297–307 (1999).
20. CÉSAR, J.A. ET AL. Impact of breastfeeding on admission for pneumonia during postneonatal period in Brazil: nested case-control study. *British medical journal,* **318**: 1316–1320 (1999).
21. TEELE, D.W. ET AL. Greater Boston Otitis Media Study Group. Epidemiology of otitis media during the first seven years of life in children in greater Boston: a prospective, cohort study. *Journal of infectious diseases,* **160**: 83–94 (1989).
22. DUNCAN, B. ET AL. Exclusive breastfeeding for at least 4 months protects against otitis media. *Pediatrics,* **91**: 867–872 (1993).
23. OWEN, M.J. ET AL. Relation of infant feeding practices, cigarette smoke exposure, and group child care to the onset and duration of otitis media

with effusion in the first two years of life. *Journal of pediatrics*, **123**: 702–711 (1993).

24. DEWEY, K.G. ET AL. Differences in morbidity between breast-fed and formula-fed infants. *Journal of pediatrics*, **126**: 696–702 (1995).

25. ANDERSSON, B. ET AL. Inhibition of attachment of *Streptococcus pneumoniae* and *Haemophilus influenzae* by human milk and receptor oligosaccharides. *Journal of infectious diseases*, **153**: 232–237 (1986).

26. COCHI, S.L. ET AL. Primary invasive *Haemophilus influenzae* type b disease: a population-based assessment of risk factors. *Journal of pediatrics*, **108**: 887–896 (1986).

27. TAKALA, A.K. ET AL. Risk factors of invasive *Haemophilus influenzae* type b disease among children in Finland. *Journal of pediatrics*, **115**: 694–701 (1989).

28. ARNON, S.S. ET AL. Protective role of human milk against sudden death from infant botulism. *Journal of pediatrics*, **100**: 568–573 (1982).

29. PISACANE, A. ET AL. Breastfeeding and urinary tract infection. *Journal of pediatrics*, **120**: 87–89 (1992).

30. HASSELBALCH, H. ET AL. Decreased thymus size in formula-fed infants compared with breast-fed infants. *Acta paediatrica*, **85**: 1029–1032 (1996).

31. HANSON, L.A. Breastfeeding provides passive and likely long-lasting active immunity. *Annals of allergy, asthma, and immunology*, **81**: 523–533 (1998).

32. GERSTEIN, H.C. Cow's milk exposure and type I diabetes mellitus. *Diabetes care*, **17**: 13–19 (1994).

33. VERGE, C.F. ET AL. Environmental factors in childhood IDDM. *Diabetes care*, **17**: 1381–1389 (1994).

34. VIRTANEN, S.M. & ARO, A. Dietary factors and the aetiology of diabetes. *Annals of medicine*, **26**: 469–478 (1994).

35. KARJALAINEN, J. ET AL. A bovine albumin peptide as a possible trigger of insulin-dependent diabetes mellitus. *New England journal of medicine*, **327**: 302–307 (1992).

36. SAUKKONEN, T. ET AL. Children with newly diagnosed IDDM have increased levels of antibodies to bovine serum albumin but not to ovalbumin. Childhood Diabetes in Finland study group. *Diabetes care*, **17**: 970–976 (1994).

37. LEVY-MARCHAL, C. ET AL. Antibodies against bovine albumin and other diabetes markers in French children. *Diabetes care*, **18**: 1089–1094 (1995).

38. RIGAS, A. ET AL. Breastfeeding and maternal smoking in the etiology of Crohn's disease and ulcerative colitis in childhood. *Annals of epidemiology*, **3**: 387–392 (1993).

39. DAVIS, M.K. Review of the evidence for an association between infant feeding and childhood cancer. *International journal of cancer,* 11 (Suppl.): 29–33 (1998).
40. SHU, X.O. ET AL. Breastfeeding and risk of childhood acute leukaemia. *Journal of the National Cancer Institute,* 91: 1765–1772 (1999).
41. VON KRIES, R. ET AL. Breastfeeding and obesity: cross sectional study. *British medical journal,* 319: 147–150 (1999).
42. BAHNA, S.L. Breast milk and special formulas in prevention of milk allergy. *Advances in experimental medicine and biology,* 310: 445–451 (1991).
43. KRAMER, M.S. Does breastfeeding help protect against atopic disease? Biology, methodology, and a golden jubilee of controversy. *Journal of pediatrics,* 112: 181–190 (1988).
44. KAY, J. ET AL. The prevalence of childhood atopic eczema in a general population. *Journal of the American Academy of Dermatology,* 30: 35–39 (1994).
45. GOLDING, J. ET AL. Eczema, asthma and allergy. *Early human development,* 49 (Suppl.): S121–S130 (1997).
46. HOFFMAN, H.J. ET AL. Risk factors for SIDS. Results of the National Institute of Child Health and Human Development SIDS Cooperative Epidemiological Study. *Annals of the New York Academy of Sciences,* 533: 13–31 (1988).
47. FORD, R.P.K. ET AL. Breastfeeding and the risk of sudden infant death syndrome. *International journal of epidemiology,* 22: 885–890 (1993).
48. ANDERSON, J.W. ET AL. Breast-feeding and cognitive development: a meta-analysis. *American journal of clinical nutrition,* 70: 525–535 (1999).
49. KENNEL, J.H. & KLAUS, M.H. Early mother-infant contact. Effects on the mother and the infant. *Bulletin of the Menninger Clinic,* 43: 69–78 (1979).
50. ARMSTRONG, H.C. Breastfeeding as the foundation of care. *Food and nutrition bulletin,* 16: 299–312 (1995).
51. ZUE, B.P. ET AL. Effect of the interval between pregnancies on perinatal outcomes. *New England journal of medicine,* 340: 589–594 (1999).
52. Consensus statement. Breastfeeding as a family planning method. *Lancet,* 2: 1204–1205 (1988).
53. KENNEDY, K.I. & VISNESS, C.M. Contraceptive efficacy of lactational amenorrhoea. *Lancet,* 339: 227–229 (1992).
54. LABBOK, M.H ET AL. The Lactational Amenorrhoea Method (LAM): a postpartum introductory family planning method with policy and program implications. *Advances in contraception,* 10: 93–109 (1994).
55. *Breastfeeding and child spacing. What health workers need to know.* Geneva, World Health Organization, 1988 (document WHO/MCH/FP/88.1).

56. DEPARTMENT OF HEALTH, UNITED KINGDOM. *Dietary reference values for food energy and nutrients for the United Kingdom. Report of the Panel on Dietary Reference Values of the Committee on Medical Aspects of Food Policy.* London, H.M. Stationery Office, 1991 (Report on Health and Social Subjects, No. 41).

57. BROWN, K.H. & DEWEY, K.G. Relationships between maternal nutritional status and milk energy output of women in developing countries. *In*: Picciano, M.F. & Lönnerdal, B., ed. *Mechanisms regulating lactation and infant nutrient utilization.* New York, Wiley-Liss, 1992, pp. 77–95.

58. *Healthy food and nutrition for women and their families. Training course and workshop curriculum for health professionals.* Copenhagen, WHO Regional Office for Europe, 2000 (document AMS 5018052).

59. *CINDI dietary guide.* Copenhagen, WHO Regional Office for Europe, 2000 (document AMS 5018028).

60. *Infant feeding in emergencies: a guide for mothers.* Copenhagen, WHO Regional Office for Europe, 1997 (document EUR/ICP/LVNG 01 02 08).

61. *Breastfeeding counselling: training course. Vol. 2. Trainer's guide.* Geneva, World Health Organization, 1993 (document WHO/CDR/93.4).

62. VINTHER, T. & HELSING, E. *Breastfeeding: how to support success. A practical guide for health workers.* Copenhagen, WHO Regional Office for Europe, 1997 (document EUR/ICP/LVNG 01 02 12).

63. PRENTICE, A. ET AL. Evidence for local feedback control of human milk secretion. *Biochemical Society transactions*, 17: 122 (1989).

64. WILDE, C.J. ET AL. Breastfeeding: matching supply with demand in human lactation. *Proceedings of the Nutrition Society*, 54: 401–406 (1995).

65. DEWEY, K.G. ET AL. WHO Working Group on Infant Growth. Growth of breast fed infants deviates from current reference data: a pooled analysis of US, Canadian, and European data sets. *Pediatrics*, 96: 495–503 (1995).

66. Resolution WHA45.34 of the Forty-fifth World Health Assembly. *In: Handbook of resolutions and decisions of the World Health Assembly and the Executive Board*, Vol. 3, 3rd ed. Geneva, World Health Organization, 1993, pp.64–66.

67. PRENTICE, A. Breast feeding and the older infant. *Acta paediatrica scandinavica*, 374 (Suppl.): 78–88 (1991).

68. BARONOWSKI, T. ET AL. Social support, social influence, ethnicity and the breastfeeding decision. *Social science and medicine*, 17: 1599–1611 (1983).

69. LIZARRAGA, J.L. ET AL. Psychosocial and economic factors associated with infant feeding intentions of adolescent mothers. *Journal of adolescent health*, 13: 676–681 (1992).

70. Entwisle, D.R. et al. Sociopsychological determinants of women's breastfeeding behavior: a replication and extension. *American journal of orthopsychiatry*, **52**: 244–260 (1982).

71. Labbok, M.H. & Simon, S.R. A community study of a decade of in-hospital breast-feeding: implications for breast-feeding promotion. *American journal of preventive medicine*, **4**: 62–66 (1988).

72. Giugliani, E.R.J. et al. Effect of breastfeeding support from different sources on mother's decisions to breastfeed. *Journal of human lactation*, **10**: 157–161 (1994).

73. *Evidence for the ten steps to successful breastfeeding.* Geneva, World Health Organization, 1998 (document WHO/CHD/98.9).

74. *International Code of Marketing of Breast-milk Substitutes.* Geneva, World Health Organization, 1981.

75. *Protecting infant health. A health worker's guide to the International Code of Marketing of Breast-milk Substitutes.* Penang, International Baby Food Action Network, 1993.

76. Commission Directive 91/321/EEC on infant formulae and follow-on formulae. *Official journal of the European Communities,* L **175**: 35 (1991).

77. Perez-Escamilla, R. et al. Determinants of lactation performance across time in an urban population from Mexico. *Social science and medicine,* **37**: 1069–1078 (1993).

78. *HIV and infant feeding.* Geneva, World Health Organization, 1998 (documents WHO/FRH/NUT 98.1, 98.2 and 98.3).

79. *Principles for evaluating health risks from chemicals during infancy and early childhood: The need for a special approach.* Geneva, World Health Organization, 1986 (Environmental Health Criteria, No. 59).

80. Grandjean, P. et al., ed. *Assessment of health risks in infants associated with exposure to PCBs, PCDDs and PCDFs in breast milk. Report on a WHO Working Group.* Copenhagen, WHO Regional Office for Europe, 1988 (document EUR/ICP/CEH 533; Environmental Health Series, No. 29).

81. US National Research Council. *Pesticides in the diets of infants and young children.* Washington, DC, National Academy Press, 1993.

82. *Breastfeeding and maternal medication.* Geneva, World Health Organization, 1995 (document WHO/CDR/95.11).

83. *Treatment of tuberculosis: guidelines for national programmes,* 2nd ed. Geneva, World Health Organization, 1997 (document WHO/TB/97.220).

84. de Martino, M. et al. Should hepatitis B surface antigen positive mothers breast feed? *Archives of disease in childhood,* **60**: 972–974 (1985).

85. SPENCER, J.D. ET AL. Transmission of hepatitis C virus to infants of human immunodeficiency virus-negative intravenous drug-using mothers: rate of infection and assessment of risk factors for transmission. *Journal of viral hepatology*, 4: 395–409 (1997).

86. KAGE, M. ET AL. Hepatitis C virus RNA present in saliva but absent in breast-milk of the hepatitis C carrier mother. *Journal of gastroenterology and hepatology*, 12: 518–521 (1997).

87. ORTEGA, R.M. ET AL. The influence of smoking on vitamin C status during the third trimester of pregnancy and on vitamin C levels in maternal milk. *Journal of the American College of Nutrition*, 17: 379–384 (1998).

88. KOTLOFF, K.L. ET AL. Diarrhoeal morbidity during the first 2 years of life among HIV-infected infants. *Journal of the American Medical Association*, 271: 448–452 (1994).

89. JOINT FAO/WHO FOOD STANDARDS PROGRAMME. *Recommended international standards for foods for infants and children*. Rome, Codex Alimentarius Commission, 1976 (CAC/RS 72/74-1976).

90. Cup feeding. *BFHI news. The Baby-Friendly Hospital Initiative newsletter*. New York, United Nations Children's Fund, May/June 1999.

91. VICTORA, C.G. ET AL. Pacifier-use and short breastfeeding duration: cause, consequence or coincidence? *Pediatrics*, 99: 445–453 (1997).

CHAPTER 8

Complementary feeding

Timely introduction of appropriate complementary foods promotes good health, nutritional status and growth of infants and young children during a period of rapid growth, and should be a high priority for public health.

Throughout the period of complementary feeding, breast-milk should continue to be the main type of milk consumed by the infant.

Complementary foods should be introduced at about 6 months of age. Some infants may need complementary foods earlier, but not before 4 months of age.

Unmodified cow's milk should not be used as a drink before the age of 9 months, but can be used in small quantities in the preparation of complementary foods from 6–9 months of age. From 9–12 months, cow's milk can be gradually introduced into the infant's diet as a drink.

Complementary foods with a low energy density can limit energy intake, and the average energy density should not usually be less than 4.2 kJ (1 kcal)/g. This energy density depends on meal frequency and can be lower if meals are offered often. Low-fat milks should not be given before the age of about 2 years.

Complementary feeding should be a process of introducing foods with an increasing variety of texture, flavour, aroma and appearance, while maintaining breastfeeding.

Highly salted foods should not be given during the complementary feeding period, nor should salt be added to food during this period.

WHAT IS COMPLEMENTARY FEEDING?

Complementary feeding is the provision of foods or fluids to infants in addition to breast-milk. Complementary foods can be subdivided into:

- transitional foods, which are complementary foods specifically designed to meet the particular nutritional or physiological needs of the infant; and

- family foods, which are complementary foods given to the young child that are broadly the same as those consumed by the rest of the family.

During the period of transition from exclusive breastfeeding to the cessation of breastfeeding, infants *gradually* become accustomed to eating family foods until they entirely replace breast-milk (see Fig. 1). Children are physically capable of consuming family foods by 1 year of age, after which they no longer need to be modified to meet the special needs of the infant.

The age during which transitional foods are introduced is a particularly sensitive time in infant development. The diet undergoes its most radical change, from a single food (breast-milk) with fat as the major energy source to one in which an increasing variety of foods are required to meet nutritional needs. This transition is associated not only with increasing and changing nutrient requirements, but also with rapid growth, physiological maturation and development of the infant.

Poor nutrition and less-than-optimum feeding practices during this critical period may increase the risk of growth faltering (wasting and stunting) and nutritional deficiencies, especially of iron, and may have longer-term adverse effects on health and mental development. Thus, nutritional interventions and improved feeding practices targeted at infants are among the most cost-effective that health professionals can promote.

PHYSIOLOGICAL DEVELOPMENT AND MATURATION

The ability to consume "solid" food requires maturation of the neuromuscular, digestive, renal and defence systems.

Neuromuscular coordination

Maturation of the neuromuscular system influences the timing of the introduction of "solid" foods and the ability of infants to consume them. Many of the feeding reflexes exhibited during the different stages of development either facilitate or interfere with the introduction of different types of food. At birth, for example, both the rooting reflex and the suck-and-swallow mechanisms facilitate breastfeeding *(1,2)* but the gag reflex may interfere with the introduction of solids.

Before 4 months, infants do not have the neuromuscular coordination to form a food bolus, transfer it to the oropharynx and swallow it. Head control and back support are immature and make it difficult for infants to maintain a position for successful ingestion and swallowing of semisolid foods. Infants start to bring objects to their mouth at about 5 months of age, and development of the "munching reflex" at this time permits consumption of some solid foods, regardless of whether or not teeth have appeared. By about 8 months, most infants can sit unsupported, their first teeth have appeared, and they have sufficient tongue flexibility to enable them to swallow thicker boluses of food. Soon after, infants have the manual skills to feed themselves, drink from a cup using two hands, and eat family foods. It is essential to encourage infants to develop eating skills, such as chewing and bringing objects to the mouth, at the appropriate stages. If these skills are not acquired early, behavioural and feeding problems may occur later on.

Some of these reflexes and age-related oral skills are listed in Table 42, together with possible implications for the types of foods that can be safely consumed. The foods mentioned in Table 42 are examples and are not the only ones that can be introduced into the diet at the different stages described. Moreover, there is no rigid relationship between food types and neurodevelopment; the infant is merely physically more capable of handling that particular food at that stage of development.

Digestion and absorption

The secretion of gastric, intestinal and pancreatic digestive enzymes is not developed to adult levels in young infants. Nevertheless, the infant is able to digest and absorb the nutrients in human milk fully and efficiently, and breast-milk contains enzymes that contribute to the hydrolysis of fat, carbohydrate and protein in the gut. Similarly, during early infancy the secretion of bile salts is only marginally adequate to permit micelle formation, and the efficiency of fat absorption is lower than in childhood and adulthood. Bile-salt-stimulated lipase, present in breast-milk but absent from commercial formulas, may in part compensate for this deficiency. By about 4 months, gastric acid assists gastric pepsin to digest protein fully.

Although pancreatic amylase begins to make an effective contribution to the digestion of starches only at the end of the first year, most cooked starches are digested and absorbed almost completely (4). Even during the first months of life, the colon plays a vital role in the final digestion of those nutrients that are not fully absorbed in the small intestine. The intracolonic microflora changes with age and in relation to whether the infant is breastfed or formula-fed. The microflora ferments undigested carbohydrates and fermentable fibre to short-chain fatty acids, which are absorbed in the colon to ensure maximum uptake of energy from carbohydrates. This process, known as "colonic salvage", may contribute up to 10% of absorbed energy.

By the time adapted family foods are introduced into the infant's diet at about 6 months, the digestive system is sufficiently mature to efficiently

Table 42. Neurological development of infants and young children and implications for types of food that can be consumed at different ages

Age (months)	Reflexes/skills present	Types of food that can be consumed[a]	Examples of foods
0–6	Suckling/sucking and swallowing	Liquids	Breast-milk
4–7	Appearance of early "munching" Increased strength of suck Movement of gag reflex from mid to posterior third of tongue	Puréed foods	Vegetable (e.g. carrot) or fruit (e.g. banana) purées; mashed potato; gluten-free cereals (e.g. rice); well cooked puréed liver and meat
7–12	Clearing spoon with lips Biting and chewing Lateral movements of tongue and movement of food to teeth	Mashed or chopped foods and finger foods	Well cooked minced liver and meat; mashed cooked vegetables and fruit; chopped raw fruit and vegetables (e.g. banana, melon, tomato); cereals (e.g. wheat, oats) and bread
12–24	Rotary chewing movements Jaw stability	Family foods	

[a] This indicates the types of food that can be consumed and swallowed successfully; it does not necessarily indicate when these foods should be offered.

Sources: Stevenson & Allaire (2); Milla (3).

digest starch, protein and fat in the non-milk diet. Nevertheless, infants have a small gastric capacity (about 30 ml/kg body weight). Thus if foods are too bulky and of low energy density, infants are sometimes unable to consume enough to satisfy their energy and nutrient requirements. Complementary foods therefore need to have a high energy and micronutrient density, and should be offered as small, frequent meals.

Renal function

Renal solute load refers to the sum of solutes that must be excreted by the kidneys. It mainly comprises nonmetabolizable dietary components, primarily the electrolytes sodium, chloride, potassium and phosphorus, which have been ingested in excess of body needs, and metabolic end-products, of which the nitrogenous compounds resulting from the digestion and metabolism of protein are the most important.

Potential renal solute load refers to solutes of dietary and endogenous origin that would have to be excreted in urine if none were diverted into the synthesis of new tissue or lost through non-renal routes. It is defined as the sum of the four electrolytes (sodium, chloride, potassium and phosphorus) plus the solutes derived from the metabolism of protein, which usually contributes more than 50% of the potential renal solute load. Table 43 shows the considerable variation in the potential renal solute load of various milks and formulas.

The newborn baby has limited renal capacity to deal with a high solute load and at the same time conserve fluids. The osmolarity of human milk is appropriate for infants and anxiety about excess renal solute load is primarily a concern for non-breastfed infants, especially those fed unmodified cow's milk. These concerns are particularly pertinent during illness. By around 4 months, renal function has matured considerably and infants can conserve water better and deal with higher solute concentrations. Thus, recommendations on complementary feeding do not ordinarily need to be modified to take account of the stage of renal development.

Defence system

The development and maintenance of an effective mucosal barrier in the intestine is an essential defence mechanism. In the neonate the mucosal barrier is immature, making it vulnerable to injury by enteropathic microorganisms and

Table 43. Potential renal solute load of various milks and formulas	
Milk or formula	Potential renal solute load (mosmol/litre)
Mature human milk	93
Commercial infant formula	135
Evaporated milk formula	260
Whole cow's milk	308

Source: Fomon *(5)*.

sensitive to some antigenic food proteins. Human milk contains a wide range of factors, absent from commercial infant formulas, that stimulate the development of active defence mechanisms and help to prepare the gastrointestinal tract for the ingestion of transitional foods. The nonimmunological defence mechanisms that help protect the intestinal surface against microorganisms, toxins and antigens include gastric acidity, mucus, intestinal secretions and peristalsis.

The relatively poor defences of the young infant's digestive tract, together with reduced gastric acidity, contribute to the risk of injury to the mucosa by foreign food and microbiological proteins, which can cause direct toxic or immunologically mediated damage. Some foods contain proteins that are potentially antigenic, such as soya protein, gluten (present in some cereals), cow's milk, egg and fish proteins, which have been associated with an enteropathy. It is therefore prudent to avoid introducing these foods before 6 months of age, particularly where there is a family history of food allergy.

WHY ARE COMPLEMENTARY FOODS NEEDED?

As the baby grows and becomes more active, breast-milk alone is insufficient to meet the full nutritional and psychological needs of the infant. Adapted family foods (transitional foods) are needed to fill the gap in energy and iron and other essential nutrients, between what is provided by exclusive breastfeeding and the total nutritional requirements of the infant (see Fig. 1). This gap increases with age, demanding an increasing contribution of energy and nutrients, especially iron, from foods other than breast-milk. Complementary foods also play an important part in the development of neuromuscular coordination.

Infants do not have the physiological maturity to progress from exclusive breastfeeding directly to family foods. Specially adapted family foods (transitional foods) are therefore necessary to bridge this gap, and are required until about 1 year of age when the infant is sufficiently mature to consume normal family foods. The introduction of transitional foods also exposes the infant to a variety of textures and consistencies, thus encouraging the development of vital motor abilities such as chewing.

WHEN SHOULD COMPLEMENTARY FOODS BE INTRODUCED?

The optimal age at which to introduce transitional foods can be determined by comparing the advantages and disadvantages of doing so at various ages.

The adequacy of breast-milk to provide sufficient energy and nutrients to maintain growth and prevent deficiencies should be assessed, together with the risk of morbidity, especially of infectious and allergic disease from contaminated foods and "foreign" food proteins. Other important considerations include physiological development and maturity, and the various developmental cues that indicate an infant's eating readiness; and maternal factors, such as nutritional status, the effect of reduced suckling on maternal fertility and caring ability and practices (see Chapter 9).

Starting complementary feeding too soon has its dangers because:

• breast-milk can be displaced by complementary foods, leading to reduced production of breast-milk and thereby the risk of insufficient energy and nutrient intake by the infant;

• infants are exposed to microbial pathogens present in foods and fluids, which are potentially contaminated and thereby increase the risk of diarrhoeal disease and consequently malnutrition;

• the risks of diarrhoeal disease and food allergies are increased because of intestinal immaturity, and these increase the risk of malnutrition; and

• mothers become fertile more quickly, because decreased suckling reduces the period during which ovulation is suppressed.

There will also be problems if complementary foods are introduced too late because:

• inadequate provision of energy and nutrients from breast-milk alone may lead to growth faltering and malnutrition;

• micronutrient deficiencies, especially of iron and zinc, may develop owing to the inability of breast-milk to meet requirements; and

• the optimal development of motor skills such as chewing, and the infant's acceptance of new tastes and textures, may not be ensured.

It is therefore necessary to introduce complementary foods at the appropriate developmental stages.

There remains much debate on when precisely to start complementary feeding. While there is agreement that the optimal age differs between individual infants, whether the recommendation should be "between 4 and 6 months" or "about 6 months" is an open question. To clarify, "6 months" is defined as the end of the first 6 months of life, when the infant is 26 weeks old, as opposed to the start of the sixth month of life, that is at 21–22 weeks of age. Likewise, "4 months" refers to the end and not the start of the fourth month of life. There is almost universal agreement that complementary feeding should not be started before the age of 4 months and should not be delayed beyond the age of 6 months. Resolutions from the World Health Assembly in 1990 and 1992 advise "4–6 months", while a 1994 resolution recommends "about 6 months". In several more recent publications from WHO and UNICEF, both expressions have been used. In a WHO review by Lutter (6) it was concluded that the scientific basis for recommending 4–6 months is not adequately documented. In a recent WHO/UNICEF report on complementary feeding in developing countries (7) the authors recommend that full-term infants should be exclusively breastfed to about 6 months of age.

The 4–6-month range is used in many recommendations from industrialized countries. In contrast, the recent official recommendations from the Netherlands (8) state that for breastfed infants with adequate growth, it is not necessary to offer any complementary food before the age of about 6 months, from a nutritional point of view. If parents decide to start earlier, however, this is acceptable provided the infant is at least 4 months old. Furthermore, a statement from the American Academy of Pediatrics (9) recommends "about six months", and various Member States in the WHO European Region also adopted this when adapting and implementing the Integrated Management of Childhood Illness (IMCI) training packages for health professionals (see Annex 3).

When deciding if the recommendation should be 4–6 or about 6 months, the way in which parents or health professionals interpret this should be assessed. Health professionals may misinterpret the recommendation and so encourage the introduction of complementary foods by 4 months, just to be "on the safe side". As a result, parents may believe that their children should be eating complementary foods by the time they reach 4 months and therefore introduce "tastes" of food before 4 months (7). National authorities should therefore assess how their recommendations are interpreted by both parents and health professionals.

In countries in economic transition, there is evidence of an increased risk of infectious disease when complementary foods are introduced before 6 months, and complementary feeding before this time does not appear to enhance the rate at which infants gain weight or length *(10,11)*. Indeed, exclusive breastfeeding for around the first 6 months confers a health advantage. In poor environmental conditions, even if energy intake increases slightly with the introduction of complementary feeding, the energy cost of reacting to the increased morbidity associated with the introduction of foods and fluids other than breast-milk (especially likely to occur in unhygienic environments) results in no net gain in terms of energy balance. For nutrients, the potential gain from the introduction of complementary foods is likely to be offset by the losses due to increased morbidity and the reduced bioavailability of nutrients from breast-milk when additional foods are given simultaneously with breast-milk. In settings where nutrient deficiency in infants under 6 months of age is a concern, improved maternal food intake may be a more effective and less risky way of preventing deficiencies in both mother and infant. Optimum maternal nutrition during pregnancy and lactation not only ensures good quality milk for the baby but also maximizes a mother's capacity to care for her infant.

For the WHO European Region, it is recommended that all infants should be exclusively breastfed from birth to about 6 months of age, and at least for the first 4 months of life. Some infants may need complementary foods before 6 months of age, but these should not be introduced before 4 months. Signs that complementary foods should be introduced before 6 months are that the baby, in the absence of obvious disease, is not gaining weight adequately (based on two or three sequential assessments) (see Chapter 10), or appears hungry after unrestricted breastfeeding. Attention should be paid to the use of appropriate growth reference charts, bearing in mind that breastfed infants have growth rates that differ from those on which the US National Center for Health Statistics references are based *(12)*. Nevertheless, consideration should also be given to other factors, including birth weight and the gestational age, clinical condition and overall growth and nutritional status of the infant when starting complementary feeding before 6 months. A study in Honduras *(13)* found that the provision of free, high-quality complementary foods from the age of 4 months to breastfed infants with a birth weight between 1500 g and 2500 g did not confer a growth advantage. These findings support the recommendation for exclusive breastfeeding for about 6 months, even in low-birth-weight infants.

COMPOSITION OF COMPLEMENTARY FOODS

In Chapter 3, estimates of the average amounts of energy required from complementary foods at different ages were defined. The effect was considered of different levels of breast-milk intake and varying energy density of complementary foods on the meal frequency required to satisfy energy requirements, taking into account the restrictions on volume dictated by gastric capacity. In the following section, these issues are revisited and explored in more detail. The physical properties of starch are discussed in relation to the thickness of the staple complementary food. Based on this, possible modifications to the preparation of the staple are proposed, which should help to produce a food that is neither too thick for the infant to consume nor so thin that energy and nutrient density are reduced. Furthermore, ways in which the nutrient density of the staple food can be improved through the addition of other complementary foods are considered, as are other factors affecting the amount of food consumed (such as flavour and aroma) and the amount of each nutrient actually absorbed (bioavailability and nutrient density).

Energy density and viscosity

The main factors influencing the extent to which an infant can meet his or her energy and nutrient requirements are the consistency and energy density (energy per unit volume) of the complementary food and the frequency of feeding. Starch often provides the principal source of energy, but when heated with water starch granules gelatinize to produce a bulky, thick (viscous) porridge. These physical properties make the porridge difficult for infants to both ingest and digest. Furthermore, the low energy and nutrient density means that large volumes of food have to be consumed to meet the infant's requirements. This is not usually possible, owing to the infant's limited gastric capacity and to the limited number of meals offered per day. Dilution of thick porridges to make them easier to swallow will further reduce their energy density. Complementary foods traditionally tend to be of low energy density and protein content, and although their liquid consistency makes them easy to consume, the volumes needed to meet infant energy and nutrient requirements often exceed the maximum volume the infant can ingest. The addition of some oil can make staples softer and easier to eat even when cold. The addition of a lot of sugar or lard, however, while improving energy density, will increase the viscosity (thickness) and therefore make the food too difficult for the infant to consume in large amounts.

Thus, complementary foods should be rich in energy, protein and micronutrients, and have a consistency that allows easy consumption. In some parts of the developing world this problem has been addressed through the addition of amylase-rich flour to thick porridges, which reduces their viscosity without reducing their energy and nutrient contents (14). Amylase-rich flour is produced by the germination of cereal grain, which activates amylase enzymes that then break down starch into sugars (maltose, maltodextrins and glucose). As starch is broken down, it loses its ability to absorb water and swell, and therefore porridge made with germinated flour rich in amylase has a high energy density while retaining a semi-liquid consistency, but increased osmolarity. These flours are time-consuming and tedious to prepare, but can be made in large quantities and added in small amounts to liquify porridges as required *(15)*. They can also be produced commercially at low cost.

Starch-containing foods can also be improved by mixing with other foods, although it is essential to be aware of the effects of such additions, not only on the viscosity of the food but also on its protein and micronutrient density. For example, while the addition of animal fats, oil or margarine increases the energy content, it has a negative effect on protein and micronutrient density. Therefore, starch-containing foods should be enriched with foods that enhance their energy, protein and micronutrient contents. This can be achieved by adding milk (breast-milk, commercial infant formula or small amounts of cow's milk or fermented milk products), which improves protein quality and increases the density of essential nutrients.

Nutrient density and bioavailability

The quantity of nutrients available for infant growth and development depends on both the amount in breast-milk and transitional foods and their bioavailability. Bioavailability is defined as the absorbability of nutrients and their availability for utilization for metabolic purposes, while nutrient density is the amount of a nutrient per unit of energy, such as 100 kJ, or per unit of weight, such as 100 g.

There are major differences between the nutrient density and bioavailability of micronutrients in animal products and plant-derived foods. Per unit of energy, animal products usually contain more of certain nutrients such as vitamins A, D and E, riboflavin, vitamin B_{12}, calcium and zinc. The iron content of some animal products (such as liver, meat, fish, and poultry) is high, whereas that of others (milk and dairy products) is low. In contrast, the densities of thiamin, vitamin B_6, folic acid and vitamin C are generally higher in plants and some, such as legumes and maize, also contain substantial amounts of iron. In general, however, the bioavailability of minerals from plant products is poor compared with that from animal products.

Micronutrients that have poor bioavailability when consumed in plant products include iron, zinc, calcium and β-carotene in leafy and some other vegetables. In addition, the absorption of β-carotene, vitamin A and other fat-soluble vitamins is impaired when diets are low in fat.

Diets with high nutrient bioavailability are diverse and contain generous amounts of legumes and foods rich in vitamin C, combined with small amounts of meat, fish and poultry. Diets with low nutrient bioavailability consist mainly of cereals, legumes and roots with negligible quantities of meat, fish or vitamin C-rich foods.

Variety, flavour and aroma

To ensure that the energy and nutrient needs of growing children are fulfilled, they should be offered a wide variety of foods of high nutritional value. Moreover, it is possible that offering children a more varied diet improves their appetite. Although patterns of food consumption vary from meal to meal, children adjust their energy intake at successive meals so that overall daily energy intake is normally relatively constant. Nevertheless, there is also some variation in energy intake from day to day. Despite having preferences, when offered a range of foods children tend to select a variety, including the preferred ones, to make a nutritionally complete diet.

A number of organoleptic features, such as flavour, aroma, appearance and texture, may affect the infant's intake of transitional foods. Taste buds detect four primary taste qualities: sweet, bitter, salt and sour. Sensitivity to taste helps protect against the ingestion of harmful substances and, in addition, can help regulate a child's intake. While children do not need to learn to like sweet or salty foods there is substantial evidence that children's preferences for the majority of other foods are strongly influenced by learning and experience (16). The only innate preference in humans is for the sweet taste, and even newborn infants avidly consume sweet substances. This can be a problem, because children develop a preference in relation to the frequency of exposure to particular tastes. Rejection of all foods except sweet ones will limit the variety of a child's intake of food and nutrients.

Children appear to consume more when they receive a varied diet compared with a monotonous one. It is important that children, for whom all foods are initially unfamiliar, have repeated exposure to new foods during the complementary feeding period in order to establish a healthy food acceptance pattern. It has been suggested that a minimum of 8–10 exposures are needed, with clear increases in food acceptance appearing after 12–15 exposures (17). Parents should thus be reassured that refusal is normal. Foods should be offered repeatedly, as those that are initially rejected are often accepted later. If the child's initial rejection is interpreted as unchangeable, the food will probably not be offered to the child again and the opportunity for exposure to new foods and tastes will be lost.

The process of complementary feeding depends on the infant learning to enjoy new foods. Breastfed infants may accept solid foods more rapidly than those fed on commercial infant formula, as they have become used to a range of flavours and odours transmitted via the mother's milk *(18)*.

PRACTICAL RECOMMENDATIONS FOR THE INTRODUCTION OF COMPLEMENTARY FOODS

The main stages in the progression of an infant's diet from breast-milk to family foods are outlined below. They make up a continuum, and transition from one to the next is relatively fast and smooth. It is essential to recognize the variations between infants in their developmental readiness for complementary feeding, and therefore individual patterns in the rate of introduction of different complementary foods. The following guidelines should help to ensure that infants receive an adequate nutrient supply, that bioavailability and nutrient density are maximized, and that appropriate behavioural skills are stimulated and developed. Chapter 9 includes a discussion of the social and domestic issues and practices that underlie successful complementary feeding.

Developmental stage 1

The aim at this initial stage is to accustom the infant to eat from a spoon. Initially only a small amount (about one or two teaspoons) of food is needed, and should be offered on the tip of a clean teaspoon or finger. It can take a little time for the baby to learn how to use the lips to clear food off a spoon, and how to move food to the back of the mouth ready for swallowing. Some food may run down the chin, or be spat out. This is to be expected at first and does not mean that the child does not like the food.

Fluids

Breastfeeding on demand should continue at the same frequency and intensity as in the period of exclusive breastfeeding, and breast-milk should remain the primary source of fluid, nutrients and energy. No other drinks are necessary at this time.

Transitional foods

The first foods offered should be single-ingredient, puréed foods with a smooth consistency, with no added sugar, salt or strong seasonings such as curry powder or chilli pepper. Good examples include non-wheat cereals such as puréed home-cooked rice, mashed potato, soft thick porridge made from traditional cereal foods such as oats, and puréed vegetables or fruit. Breast-milk (or infant formula) can be added to purées to help soften them.

Meal frequency

Small amounts of complementary foods once or twice a day will help the baby to learn the skill of eating food and enjoying new tastes. Foods should be offered after breastfeeding in order to avoid replacing breast-milk.

Developmental stage 2

Once the infant has accepted spoon feeding, new tastes and textures can be added to increase the variety of the diet and to help the development of motor skills (Table 42). Developmental cues that infants are ready for thicker purées include their ability to sit without support and to transfer objects from one hand to the other.

Fluids

Breastfeeding on demand should continue, and breast-milk should remain the primary source of fluid, nutrients and energy. The infant may not maintain the same frequency and intensity of breastfeeding as during exclusive breastfeeding.

Transitional foods

Well cooked puréed meat (especially liver), pulses, vegetables, fruit and different cereals can be introduced. To encourage infants to accept new foods, it is a good idea to introduce a new flavour, such as meat, with a familiar favourite such as puréed fruit or vegetables. Similarly, when introducing lumpier foods, a familiar favourite of the infant's should be mixed with the new, coarser-textured food (such as carrots with small, noticeable lumps). Savoury foods should be encouraged rather than sweet ones, and desserts should be low in sugar.

Meal frequency

A few weeks into the complementary feeding period, infants should be having between two and three small meals a day, selected from a wide variety of foods.

Developmental stage 3

As infants continue to develop, foods with a thicker consistency and a lumpier texture can be introduced to help them learn to chew and manage small pieces of food. With the development of fine motor skills and the appearance of teeth, infants are able to pick up small pieces of food, transfer them to the mouth and chew them; it is important to encourage these skills by offering finger foods.

Fluids

Breastfeeding on demand should continue to ensure a constant energy intake from breast-milk. As the infant grows, however, the energy and nutrients from transitional foods become increasingly important to ensure that the infant's growing nutrient requirements are met. Cow's milk and other milk products can be used in small amounts in the preparation of foods, and after 9 months unmodified cow's milk can be given as a drink to infants who are no longer breastfed. Fluids other than breast-milk should be given in a cup.

Transitional foods

Vegetables need to be cooked until soft, and meats should be minced and then coarsely puréed. Meals should be varied and contain fruit and vegetables, legumes and small amounts of fish, kefir, meat, liver, egg or cheese. To prevent the risk of salmonella poisoning, it is essential to cook eggs well; dishes containing raw eggs should not be used (see Chapter 12). Finger foods such as toasted bread, carrot and pear should be offered at each meal. Moderate amounts of butter or margarine should be used on bread, while foods with added sugar such as biscuits and cakes should be discouraged.

Meal frequency

Two or three main meals should be offered each day, and can be interspersed with snacks such as yoghurt, small amounts of kefir, mashed raw or stewed apple, and bread spread with butter or margarine or jam. Infants who are not breastfed or formula-fed will need at least five meals a day by this stage.

Developmental stage 4

During the latter months of the complementary feeding period, feeding of the infant should be combined with self-feeding. While infants and young children practise their feeding skills, however, they cannot self-feed enough to achieve adequate intake and caregivers still have an active role in feeding (Chapter 9).

Fluids

Breast-milk continues to be an important part of the diet and should preferably be the main fluid into the second year and beyond. The intake of fresh cow's milk and cow's milk products can be gradually increased from the age of 9 months.

Transitional foods

As the infant progresses to a more mature diet, foods should be chopped or mashed, and meat should be minced. Finger foods, such as small cubes of fruit, vegetables, potato, toast, cheese and soft meat, should be included at each meal to encourage the infant to feed himself or herself. Feeds made up of high-fat foods alone should be avoided.

Meal frequency

Infants should receive three main meals interspersed with about two snacks per day.

By the age of about 1 year, children can share the normal family diet and do not require specially prepared foods. Adding salt is still not recommended, and its restriction will benefit the whole family. Children eat slowly, so special considerations have to be made to allow for the extra time and attention needed (Chapter 9). Infants and young children need encouragement when learning to eat, and the adults who feed them need patience. Helping and encouraging toddlers to eat, rather than leaving them to serve themselves from the family dish, can greatly increase the amount of food they consume. Infants and young children should always be supervised during feeding (Chapter 9).

WHAT ARE THE BEST FOODS TO PREPARE FOR INFANTS?

The choice of foods used for complementary feeding differs considerably between populations, owing to tradition and availability. The following section discusses the use of different foods for complementary feeding. A useful way of calculating the contribution of different foods to fill the energy and nutrient gap left when breast-milk no longer meets the infant's growing needs is given in a new WHO report *(19)*.

Foods of plant origin

Food contains combinations of other substances in addition to nutrients, most of which are abundant in plants. No single food can supply every nutrient (with the exception of breast-milk for young infants). For example, potatoes provide vitamin C but do not provide iron, while bread and dried beans provide iron but not vitamin C. To prevent disease and promote growth, a healthy diet must therefore contain a variety of foods.

Plant foods contain biologically active components or metabolites that have been used for centuries in traditional cures and herbal medicines. The isolation, identification and quantification of these plant metabolites is related to their potential protective role, and interest in identifying them has arisen because of the epidemiological evidence showing that some protect against cancer and cardiovascular disease in adults. It is plausible that such components also have beneficial effects on young children, although scientific evidence is lacking. Many plant metabolites are not nutrients in the traditional sense and are sometimes called "non-nutrients". They include substances such as dietary fibre and related substances, phytosterols, lignans, flavonoids, glucosinolates, phenols, terpenes and allium compounds. These are found in a variety of different plants, some of which are listed in Table 44.

To ensure an intake of all these protective substances, it is important to eat as wide a variety of different plant foods as possible. Taking vitamin supplements or extracted plant substances as a replacement for, or in addition to, eating good wholesome food is unnecessary and is generally not recommended on health grounds.

Cereals

Cereals form the staple foods of virtually all populations. Those that contribute significantly to the diet in the WHO European Region are wheat, buckwheat, barley, rye, oats and rice. In general, cereals contain 65–75% of their total weight as carbohydrate, 6–12% as protein and 1–5% as fat. The majority of the carbohydrate is present as starch, but cereals are also a major source of fibre and contain some simple sugars. Most raw cereals contain slowly digestible starch, which becomes rapidly digested when cooked. Partially milled grains and seeds contain starch resistant to digestion.

Cereals are also a source of micronutrients. These are concentrated in the outer bran layers of the cereal grain, which also contain phytates that can have a negative effect on the absorption of several micronutrients. Thus the high-extraction flours such as wholemeal flour, which contain more of the outer layers of the grain, are richer in micronutrients but also contain a higher proportion of phytates. Conversely the finer, whiter flours, which have a smaller proportion of the original grain, have a lower phytate content but are also lower in micronutrients.

Table 44. Examples of "non-nutrients" and their plant food sources	
"Non-nutrient"	Plant food source
Fibre and related substances	Oats, wheat, rye, soyabean, most vegetables and fruit
Phytosterols	Maize, rape seed, sunflower seed, soya bean
Lignans	Rye bran, berries, nuts
Flavonoids	Onion, lettuce, tomato, peppers, citrus fruits, soya products
Glucosinolates	Broccoli, cabbage, brussels sprouts
Phenols	Grapes, raspberries, strawberries
Terpenes	Citrus fruits, cherries, herbs
Allium compounds	Garlic, onion, leek

Potatoes

The potato is a stem tuber and a major constituent of the diet in many European countries. Potatoes are rich in starch and because they can be stored under simple conditions for quite long periods, together with cereals they offer a staple supply of food energy throughout the year. Potatoes contain relatively little protein, although the biological value of potato protein is quite high. Potatoes contain significant amounts of vitamin C and are also a good source of thiamin. The content of vitamin C in potatoes varies with length of storage: approximately two thirds of the ascorbic acid remains after 3 months and about one third remains after 6–7 months. Freshly cooked potato is rapidly and easily digestible. If it is cooled after cooking, however, its starch may become retrograded, forming so-called "resistant starch" that is indigestible in the small intestine though fermentable in the colon.

Vegetables and fruit

Vegetables and fruit provide vitamins, minerals, starch and fibre, together with other non-nutrient substances such as antioxidants and phytosterols (see above). They play a major protective role, helping to prevent micronutrient deficiency, and generally have a low fat content.

Vegetables and fruit make the most significant contribution to vitamin C intake. Eating vegetables and fruit that contain vitamin C (for example cabbage, broccoli, and the citrus fruits and their juices), along with iron rich foods such as beans, lentils and whole-grain cereals, will improve the absorption of non-haem iron from plant foods (see Chapter 6). Other micronutrients present in vegetables and fruits are the B vitamins, including vitamin B_6. Dark-green leaves and orange-coloured fruits and vegetables are rich in carotenoids, which are converted to vitamin A, and dark-green leaves are also rich in folate, with potassium and magnesium present in significant levels.

Vegetables and fruits contain different vitamins, minerals, non-nutrients (such as antioxidants) and fibre, and it is therefore advisable to choose a variety to meet daily nutrient recommendations. Some of the health benefits associated with vegetables and fruits may come from non-nutrient components. This is one reason why vitamins and minerals are best obtained from vegetables and fruit rather than from tablets or supplements, ensuring that other (perhaps as yet undiscovered) essential food constituents are also eaten.

The availability of fresh vegetables and fruit varies by season and region, although frozen, dried and preserved vegetables and fruits can ensure a supply of these foods throughout the year. Wherever possible, locally grown produce should be selected. If they are preserved, or if processed products are used, they should contain the minimum possible amounts of added fats, oils, sugars and salt.

Many green leafy vegetables are cooked before consumption. Cooking in water can lead to leaching and thermal losses of vitamin C, especially when the vegetables are left to stand before consumption. Using only a minimum amount of water, or boiling for a very short time, reduces vitamin losses.

Legumes

Legumes, and particularly seed legumes (soya beans, peas, beans and lentils), are of major nutritional value, particularly when animal products are scarce. They have a low water content when mature, store well, and in many diets are an important source of nutrients when eaten alongside cereals. The seed legumes have a high protein content and the protein is of good biological value. The seeds are rich in complex carbohydrates, both starch and dietary fibre, and they also provide significant quantities of vitamins and minerals.

Some legumes, however, contain a range of toxic constituents including lectins, which act as haemagglutinins and trypsin inhibitors. When mature, a number of seeds (such as kidney bean) contain toxic concentrations of these constituents, and it is therefore vital that they are prepared correctly, with thorough soaking and cooking, to avoid any toxic effect.

Foods of animal origin

Animal products are rich sources of protein, vitamin A and easily absorbable iron and folate. Meat and fish are the best sources of zinc, while dairy products are rich in calcium. Meat, fish and seafood all promote the absorption of non-haem iron, and meat (especially liver and other offal) also provide well absorbed haem iron (Chapter 6). Epidemiological studies have shown that meat consumption is associated with a lower prevalence of iron deficiency. Animal products, however, are often expensive and eating excess protein is uneconomic and inefficient as the extra protein will be broken down into energy and stored as fat if the energy is not immediately required. If it is energy that is needed, it is more efficient to obtain it from energy-dense foods rich in micronutrients rather than from protein.

Meat

Nutrients are present in different concentrations in the fat and lean tissues of meat, being more concentrated in the lean tissue. The ratio of fat to lean tissue therefore determines the energy value and the concentration of nearly all nutrients. In western Europe, current nutritional advice to the general population is to reduce saturated fat intake, and leaner carcasses are now in demand. In contrast, in central and eastern parts of the Region, the fat content of most meats and meat products is still very high. Liver, however, is naturally low in fat and has the additional benefit of being easily cooked and puréed without becoming stringy, and is thus easier for infants and young children to eat. Indeed, liver deserves a special mention as one of the best transitional foods, since it is an excellent source of protein and of most essential micronutrients.

Lean meat contains substantial amounts of protein of high biological value, and is an important source of highly bioavailable minerals such as iron and zinc. Young children may have difficulty eating meat because of its stringy nature, and meat (preferably lean) used in complementary foods should be minced, chopped or puréed.

Even though some meats are expensive, some (such as liver) are not, and only small amounts can have nutritional benefits in infants and young children. Small amounts of meat added to an otherwise vegetarian diet have a positive effect on length gain *(20,21)*, either through the better biological value of the protein or because of the minerals provided.

Fish and seafood

Fish is an important source of good quality protein, weight-for-weight providing the same quantities as lean meat. Moreover all fish, both freshwater and saltwater fish and shellfish, are rich sources of essential amino acids. This protein is accompanied by very low amounts of fat in white fish and shellfish, while the fat in other fish (such as salmon, tuna, sardines, herring and mackerel) has a high proportion of n-3 long-chain polyunsaturated fatty acids, which are important for neurodevelopment. Fish represents a good source of iron and zinc, which are found in slightly lower concentrations than in meat with the exception of shellfish, which tend to accumulate trace elements. Oysters, for example, are one of the richest sources of zinc. Saltwater fish are also a key source of iodine, which is accumulated from their marine environment. Care is needed because of the potential risks of eating fish caught in water that is contaminated (see Chapter 12).

Eggs

The eggs of a range of domesticated birds, including chickens, ducks and geese, are important in the diet throughout the European Region. Eggs provide a versatile food of high biological value. Egg proteins contain amino acids essential to growth and development, and the lipids in eggs are rich in phospholipids with a high ratio of polyunsaturated to saturated fatty acids. Eggs can be produced efficiently and relatively cheaply, and are a valuable means of improving the intake of animal protein. Egg protein has been associated with allergic reactions and should therefore not be introduced before the age of 6 months. Eggs are a potential cause of salmonella poisoning (see Chapter 12) and so should be thoroughly cooked.

Eggs are often thought of as a good source of iron, and as a result are introduced early into the complementary diet. Although their iron content is relatively high, however, the iron is bound to phosphoprotein and albumin and is therefore not very bioavailable.

Milk and other dairy products

The nutritional composition of fresh cow's milk makes it a source of many nutrients for the growing child, but it should not be introduced before the age of 9 months (Chapter 6) because:

- it may displace breast-milk intake;
- it has a low iron content;
- it may cause gastrointestinal bleeding, especially before the age of 6 months; and
- it has a high protein and sodium content, 3–4 times greater than that of human milk.

To ensure that animal milks are microbiologically safe, it is important that they are either pasteurized or boiled before consumption (Chapter 12). Cow's milk from which the fat has been partly (semi-skimmed milk, usually 1.5–2% fat) or fully (skimmed milk, usually < 0.5% fat) removed has a significantly lower energy and fat-soluble vitamin content than whole cow's milk. Similarly, powdered milks made from dried, skimmed milk have a low energy content. Furthermore, like commercial infant formula, powdered milks may become contaminated if they are made up with unclean water. It is therefore essential to prepare them under hygienic conditions, strictly following instructions to ensure that the reconstituted milk is neither too concentrated nor too dilute.

Lactose intolerance (due to loss of expression of intestinal lactase in children in some nonpastoral populations) is rare in the European Region, and does not represent a contraindication to the use of cow's milk or the milk of other mammals during complementary feeding.

Age of introduction of cow's milk

Some mothers may be unable to provide sufficient breast-milk during late infancy to satisfy their infant's requirement. This can be for a variety of reasons, including the need or choice to return to work. Some countries recommend that cow's milk is excluded from the infant's diet until the age of 12 months. Before 12 months, they recommend that infants are given breast-milk only, or commercial infant formula, primarily for the reasons listed above. Other countries recommend that cow's milk can gradually be introduced from the age of 9 or 10 months. There are no negative effects of giving breast-milk or commercial infant formula up to the age of 12 months, provided sufficient amounts are given and the iron content of complementary foods is adequate. In many countries in the Region, however, commercial infant formula is much more expensive than cow's milk, and therefore giving commercial infant formula to 12 months of age may be economically prohibitive. Based on these arguments, it is prudent to make the following recommendations for the optimal time of introduction of cow's milk.

Unmodified cow's milk should not be used as a drink, and milk products should not be given in large quantities, before the age of 9 months. They can, however, be used in small quantities in the preparation of complementary foods from the age of 6 months. Between 9 and 12 months of age, cow's milk and other milk products given as a drink can be gradually introduced into the infant's diet, preferably in addition to breast-milk, if breast-milk intake is not sufficient or if the family wants to change from infant formula.

Amount of cow's milk

It is recommended that breastfeeding should continue throughout the first year of life and into the second year if possible. If the volume of breast-milk is still high (more than about 500 ml per day) there is no reason to introduce other milks. Nevertheless, many women in the Region stop breastfeeding before their baby is 1 year of age, and if they continue to breastfeed during the 9–12-month period the average milk intake is low. If the total milk intake is very low or nil, there is a risk of deficiency of several nutrients, and potentially a problem with protein quality if there are no other sources of animal protein. During late infancy (from about 9 months) an excessive intake of cow's milk could limit diversification of the diet, which is important in exposing the infant to new tastes and textures that promote the development of eating skills. Furthermore, because the content and bioavailability of iron in cow's milk is low, a large intake predisposes an infant to iron deficiency. For example, if a 12-month-old infant consumes one litre of cow's milk or the equivalent in milk products, as much as two thirds of his or her energy requirement are covered, leaving very little room for a varied healthy diet.

Low-fat milks

In many countries, milk with a reduced fat content is recommended for adults as part of a healthy diet. It is not recommended before the age of 1 year, however, and in some countries not before 2–3 years of age. In the United Kingdom, for example, semi-skimmed milk is not normally recommended before the age of 2 years, and fully skimmed milk is not recommended until the child is over 5 years old (17). The recommendation to delay the introduction of fat-reduced milks is not only because of their low energy density but also because protein constitutes a considerably higher proportion of their energy. In skimmed milk, for example, protein constitutes 35% of energy compared to 20% in full fat milk and only 5% in breast-milk. If a large proportion of the energy intake comes from fat-reduced milks, this will increase the protein intake to levels that may be harmful. On the other hand, fat-reduced milk is not harmful if given in small to moderate amounts, and if additional fat is added to the diet.

Thus it is prudent not to introduce fat-reduced milks before the age of about 2 years. When introducing other milks, such as goat's, sheep's, camel's and mare's milk, into the infant's diet, the same basic guidelines should be followed. Allowances should be made for the varying solute loads and vitamin and mineral contents of different milks, and in all cases it is vital to ensure that they are microbiologically safe.

Fermented milk products

Liquid milk has a short shelf life. Fermentation extends its shelf life and thereby allows milk and its products to be stored and transported. Most fermented milks are the product of fermentation with lactobacilli, which leads to the generation of lactic and short-chain fatty acids from lactose, and consequently a fall in pH that inhibits the growth of many pathogenic microorganisms. Fermented milks are nutritionally similar to unfermented milk, except that some of the lactose is broken down to glucose, galactose and the products described above. These fermented milks represent an excellent source of nutrients such as calcium, protein, phosphorus and riboflavin.

A number of health benefits have traditionally been attributed to fermented milk products, and they have been used to prevent a wide range of diseases including atherosclerosis, allergies, gastrointestinal disorders and cancer *(22)*. Although empirical findings are yet to be supported by controlled studies, initial results from investigations into the antibacterial, immunological, antitumoral and hypocholesterolaemic effects of fermented milk consumption suggest potential benefits. In young children there is increasing evidence that certain strains of lactobacilli have a beneficial effect against the occurrence and duration of acute diarrhoea *(23)*. The potential health effects, also called probiotic effects, are caused by either the large amount of live bacteria present in the product, or by short-chain fatty acids or other substances produced during fermentation.

Fermented milk products are thought to enhance the absorption of non-haem iron, as a result of their lower pH. The two most common fermented milks available in the Region that contain probiotics are yoghurt and kefir.

Yoghurt is produced when milk (usually cow's milk) is fermented with *Lactobacillus bulgaricus* and *Streptococcus thermophilus* under defined conditions of time and temperature.

Kefir is a fermented milk with a characteristic fizzy, acidic taste, which originated in the Caucasus mountains and currently accounts for 70% of the total amount of fermented milk consumed in the countries of the former Soviet Union *(24)*. It is produced when kefir grains (small clusters of microorganisms held together in a polysaccharide matrix) or mother cultures prepared from the grains are added to milk and cause its fermentation.

Cheese is also a fermented milk product, in which the unstable liquid is converted into a concentrated food that can be stored. Hard cheeses are approximately one third protein, one third fat and one third water, and are also rich sources of calcium, sodium and vitamin A and, to a lesser extent, the B vitamins. Soft cheeses such as cottage cheese contain more water than hard cheese and are therefore less nutrient- and energy-dense. Cubed or diced cheese can be introduced in small amounts into the complementary feeding diet at around 6–9 months of age, but the intake of cheese spreads should be limited before 9 months.

Fruit juices

In this publication, fruit juice refers to the juice produced by compressing fruits. The term fruit juice or fruit drink is sometimes used to describe a drink made from jam or compote mixed with water. These usually contain only water and sugar, with negligible vitamin C, and therefore have none of the benefits of "real" fruit juice or the fruits from which juice can be made.

Nutritionally, fruit juices produced from compressed fruit contain all the nutrients present in fruits with the exception of the dietary fibre. The major sources are citrus fruits such as orange, lemon and grapefruit. Apple and grape juice are also common, and in Europe fruit nectars such as those made from apricot, pear and peach are also popular. Fruit juices are a good source of vitamin C, and if given as part of a meal will improve the bioavailability of non-haem iron present in plant foods. It is nevertheless important to limit the volume given to avoid interfering with the intake of breast-milk and with the diversification of the diet. Furthermore, fruit juices contain glucose, fructose, sucrose or other sugars, which because of their acidity can cause dental caries and erosion of the teeth.

In some populations there is a belief that fruit juice should not be given to infants because it is too acid, and tea is given instead. While it is true that some fruit juices have a very low pH, there is no logical reason to avoid giving them to infants or to recommend tea in preference. The pH of the stomach is close to 1 (very acidic) and acidic fruit juices have no adverse effects. However, there are concerns raised by the extreme consumption of so-called fruit juices containing artificial sweeteners and simple carbohydrates other than glucose, sucrose or fructose. Those containing sugar alcohols, such as mannitol and sorbitol, have been blamed for diarrhoea in some children *(25,26)*.

Honey

Honey may contain the spores of *Clostridium botulinum*, the causal agent of botulism. Since the gastrointestinal tract of infants contains insufficient acid to kill these spores, honey should not be given to infants lest they contract the disease.

Tea

Tea is a popular drink throughout the European Region but is not recommended for infants and young children. Tea contains tannins and other compounds that bind iron and other minerals, thereby reducing their bioavailability. Furthermore, sugar is often added, which increases the risk of dental caries. Also, sugar consumed in tea may blunt the appetite and inhibit the consumption of more nutrient-dense foods.

Herbal teas

In many western European countries, there is a growing trend towards the use of "natural" substances and alternative medicines, and this has led to an increase in the use of herbal preparations for infants. Owing to their small size and rapid growth rate, however, infants are potentially more vulnerable than adults to the pharmacological effects of some of the chemical substances present in herbal teas. Herbal teas such as camomile tea may also have the same adverse effects on non-haem iron absorption as other teas including green tea (27). There is moreover a lack of scientific data on the safety of various herbs and herbal teas for infants.

Vegetarian and vegan diets

Vegetarian diets exclude, to various degrees, animal products. The main area of concern regarding vegetarian diets is the small but significant risk of nutritional deficiencies. These include deficiencies of iron, zinc, riboflavin, vitamin B_{12}, vitamin D and calcium (especially in vegans) and inadequate energy intake. These deficiencies are highest in those with increased requirements, such as infants, children and pregnant and lactating women. Although the inclusion of animal products does not ensure the adequacy of a diet, it is easier to select a balanced diet with animal products than without them. Meat and fish are important sources of protein, readily absorbed haem iron, zinc, thiamin, riboflavin, niacin and vitamins A and B_{12}. In a vegetarian diet, these nutrients must come from other sources.

Eggs, cheese and milk all provide high-quality protein and are also a good source of the B group vitamins and calcium. Problems may occur as a result of complementary diets containing no animal products (and thereby no milk), particularly during late infancy and early childhood when the breast-milk supply may be low. Such diets rely solely on plant proteins, and the only plant protein approaching the quality of animal protein comes from soya. If it is not prepared correctly, however, feeding soya during infancy has potential negative effects because of its high content of phyto-estrogens and antinutrients such as phytate. It may also evoke antigenic reactions, and can cause an enteropathy similar to that of coeliac disease and cow's milk protein intolerance. The protein of the vegan diet must be made up of a good *mix* of plant proteins, such as legumes accompanied by wheat, or rice with lentils. For adults, protein from two or more plant groups daily is likely to be adequate. For children, however, and especially those aged 6–24 months, each meal should contain wherever possible two complementary sources of plant protein.

Vegan diets (those with no source of animal protein and especially no milk) may have serious adverse effects on infant development and should be discouraged. Examples are very restrictive macrobiotic diets (a restrictive vegetarian regimen coupled with adherence to natural and organic foods, especially cereals), which carry a high risk of nutrient deficiencies and have been associated with protein–energy malnutrition, rickets, growth retardation and delayed psychomotor development in infants and children *(28,29)*. Such diets are not recommended during the complementary feeding period *(30)*.

SOME PRACTICAL RECOMMENDATIONS FOR FOOD PREPARATION

Family foods

Home-prepared foods usually provide a sound foundation for complementary feeding and their use is encouraged. A good start to complementary feeding is to use a mixture of family foods, with the staple food (such as bread, potato, rice or buckwheat) as a base. A wide variety of household foods can be used. Most need to be softened by cooking and then puréed, mashed or chopped. A small amount of breast-milk or cooled boiled water may need to be added when puréeing food, but not so that the food is too dilute and no longer nutrient-dense. Transitional foods should be relatively bland and not strongly seasoned with either salt or sugar. Only minimal amounts of sugar should be added to sour fruits to improve their palatability. Adding unnecessary extra sugar to infant foods and drinks may encourage a preference for sweet foods later in life, with adverse effects on dental and general health (see Chapter 11).

Ideally, infants should share family meals. The foods they receive should be prepared, as far as possible, without added sugar or salt. Very salty foods such as pickled vegetables and salted meats should be avoided. A portion of family food should be removed for the infant, and flavourings such as salt or spices can then be added for the rest of the family.

As discussed above, some complementary foods have a low energy and nutrient density or can be bulky and viscous, making them difficult for an infant to consume. Conversely, gruels and soups that are easy for the infant to eat cannot be consumed in the volumes necessary to meet the infant's nutritional requirements. To improve the nutritional quality and energy density of porridges and other bulky foods, therefore, caregivers should:

- cook with less water and make a thicker porridge;
- replace most (or all) water with breast-milk or formula milk;

- enrich thick porridge by adding, for example, milk powder, oil or fat (not more than one teaspoon per 100 g serving, to avoid excess) but restrict the use of sugars, which are not so energy-dense as oils and fats;
- add fruit or vegetables rich in micronutrients; and
- add a little protein-rich food such as kefir, eggs, legumes, liver, meat or fish.

Caregivers should choose suitable foods and cook them in a way that maximizes their nutritional value. Feeding guidelines should be available to all caregivers to help them know what and how to feed their children. Education about infant feeding, as with breastfeeding, should begin at school and should be included in antenatal classes and after the birth of the baby, and be provided by primary health care staff including health visitors.

Commercial baby foods

Commercial baby foods can be convenient but are often expensive and may offer no nutritional advantages over properly prepared family foods, except where there is a special need for micronutrient fortification. Even if caregivers decide to feed commercially prepared infant foods, home-prepared foods should also be given to accustom the infant to a greater range of flavours and textures.

Policy-makers should refer to the recommendations of the Codex Alimentarius Commission *(31)*, a report jointly sponsored by WHO and FAO that specifies compositional standards for commercial baby foods. Many countries in economic transition represent a new market for baby food companies, and some lack the means of regulating the marketing, quality and composition of commercially produced infant feeds. Although commercial baby foods are popular with parents because they are quick, easy and convenient to prepare, these advantages need to be balanced against the relative cost, which may be prohibitive for low-income families.

REFERENCES

1. SHEPPARD, J.J. & MYSAK, E.D. Ontogeny of infantile oral reflexes and emerging chewing. *Child development,* 55: 831–843 (1984).
2. STEVENSON, R.D. & ALLAIRE, J.H. The development of normal feeding and swallowing. *Pediatric clinics of North America,* 38: 1439–1453 (1991).
3. MILLA, P.J. Feeding, tasting, and sucking. *In: Pediatric gastrointestinal disease. Vol. 1.* Philadelphia, B.C. Decker, 1991, pp. 217–223.

4. DE VIZIA, B. ET AL. Digestibility of starches in infants and children. *Journal of pediatrics*, **86**: 50–55 (1975).

5. FOMON, S.J. Water and renal solute load. *In*: Fomon, S.J. *Nutrition of normal infants*. St Louis, MO, Mosby, 1993.

6. LUTTER, C. *Recommended length of exclusive breastfeeding, age of introduction of complementary foods and the weaning dilemma.* Geneva, World Health Organization, 1992 (document WHO/CDD/EDP/92.5).

7. *Complementary feeding of young children in developing countries: a review of current scientific knowledge.* Geneva, World Health Organization, 1998 (document WHO/NUT/98.1).

8. *Feeding of young children: starting points for advice on feeding of children aged 0–4 years.* The Hague, Health Care Inspectorate and Nutrition Centre, 1999.

9. AMERICAN ACADEMY OF PEDIATRICS. Working Group on Breastfeeding. Breastfeeding and the use of human milk. *Pediatrics*, **100**: 1035–1039 (1997).

10. COHEN, R.J. ET AL. Effects of age of introduction of complementary foods on infant breast milk intake, total energy intake, and growth: a randomised intervention study in Honduras. *Lancet*, **344**: 288–293 (1994).

11. COHEN, R.J. ET AL. Determinants of growth from birth to 12 months among breast-fed Honduran infants in relation to age of introduction of complementary foods. *Pediatrics*, **96**: 504–510 (1995).

12. WHO WORKING GROUP ON INFANT GROWTH. *An evaluation of infant growth. A summary of analyses performed in preparation for the WHO Expert Committee on Physical Status: the use and interpretation of anthropometry.* Geneva, World Health Organization, 1994 (document WHO/NUT/94.8).

13. DEWEY, K.G. ET AL. Age of introduction of complementary foods and growth of term, low birth weight breast-fed infants: a randomised intervention study in Honduras. *American journal of clinical nutrition*, **69**: 679–686 (1999).

14. WEAVER, L.T. Feeding the weanling in the developing world: problems and solutions. *International journal of food sciences and nutrition*, **45**: 127–134 (1994).

15. WALKER, A.F & PAVITT, F. Energy density of Third World weaning foods. *British Nutrition Foundation nutrition bulletin*, **14**: 88–101 (1989).

16. BIRCH, L. Development of food acceptance patterns in the first years of life. *Proceedings of the Nutrition Society,* **57**: 617–624 (1998).

17. SULLIVAN, S.A. & BIRCH, L.L. Infant dietary experience and acceptance of solid foods. *Pediatrics*, **93**: 271–277 (1994).

18. DEPARTMENT OF HEALTH, UNITED KINGDOM. *Weaning and the weaning diet. Report of the Working Group on the Weaning Diet of the Committee on Medical Aspects of Food Policy.* London, H.M. Stationery Office, 1994 (Report on Health and Social Subjects, No. 45).

19. *Complementary feeding. Family foods for breastfed children.* Geneva, World Health Organization, 2000 (document WHO/NHD/00.1; WHO/FCH/CAH/00.6).

20. ALLEN, L.H. Nutritional influences on linear growth: a general review. *European journal of clinical nutrition*, 48 (Suppl. 1): S75–S89 (1994).

21. GOLDEN, M.H.N. Is complete catch-up possible for stunted malnourished children? *European journal of clinical nutrition*, 48 (Suppl. 1): S58–S71 (1994).

22. MACFARLANE, G.T. & CUMMINGS, J.H. Probiotics and prebiotics: can regulating the activities of intestinal bacteria benefit health? *British medical journal*, 318: 999–1003 (1999).

23. SAAVEDRA, J. Probiotics and infectious diarrhea. *American journal of gastroenterology*, 95 (Suppl. 1): S16–S18 (2000).

24. KOMAI, M. & NANNO, M. Intestinal microflora and longevity. *In*: Nakazawa, Y. & Hosono, A. *Functions of fermented milk.* London, Elsevier Applied Science, 1992, p.343.

25. LIFSHITZ, F. & AMENT, M.E. Role of juice carbohydrate malabsorption in chronic non-specific diarrhoea in children. *Journal of pediatrics*, 120: 825–829 (1992).

26. HOURIHANE, J.O. & ROLLES, C.J. Morbidity from excessive intake of high energy fluids: the "squash drinking syndrome". *Archives of disease in childhood*, 72: 141–143 (1995).

27. AHMAD, N. & MUKHTAR, H. Green tea polyphenols and cancer: biologic mechanisms and practical implications. *Nutrition reviews*, 57: 78–83 (1999).

28. DAGNELIE, P.C. ET AL. Nutritional status of infants aged 4–18 months on macrobiotic diets and matched omnivorous control infants: a population-based mixed longitudinal study. II. Growth and psychomotor development. *European journal of clinical nutrition*, 43: 325–338 (1989).

29. TRUESDELL, D.D. & ACOSTA, P.B. Feeding the vegan infant and child. *Journal of the American Dietetic Association*, 85: 837–840 (1985).

30. JACOBS, C. & DWYER, J.T. Vegetarian children: appropriate and inappropriate diets. *American journal of clinical nutrition*, 48: 811–818 (1988).

31. JOINT FAO/WHO CODEX ALIMENTARIUS COMMISSION. *Codex alimentarius.* Rome, Food and Agriculture Organization of the United Nations, 1992.

CHAPTER 9

Caring practices

Policy-makers and health professionals should recognize the need to support caregivers, and the fact that caring practices and resources for care are fundamental determinants of good nutrition and feeding and thereby of child health and development.

INTRODUCTION

Care refers to the provision (in both the household and the community) of time, attention and support to meet the physical, mental and social needs of the growing child and other household members *(1)*. It should be distinguished from "caring capacity", which describes the *potential* of a family or community to provide care but does not say whether the care is actually provided. From the information summarized in Chapter 1 it is clear that poor nutrition often results from poor feeding practices, which are prevalent throughout the European Region. Caring practices may not be optimal, and resources for adequate care at community and government levels may be insufficient.

Caring practices and resources for care (human, economic and organizational – see below) may not receive much attention by policy-makers and health professionals, perhaps because daily, time-consuming and routine activities, primarily performed by women, are not seen as critical to child health. Yet caring practices can have a lasting effect on a child's life. The ways in which caring practices are performed – with affection and with responsiveness to children – are crucial to their growth and development.

THE UNICEF CARE INITIATIVE AND NUTRITION

The immediate determinants of good nutrition, child health and survival are dietary intake and health. However, as Fig. 16 illustrates, caregiving behaviour has a direct impact on the nutrient intake and thereby the health of the child. Food, health and care must *all* be satisfactory for good nutrition. Breastfeeding is an example of a practice that provides all of these simultaneously. Even when poverty results in a lack of food and limited health care, enhanced caregiving can optimize the use of existing resources to promote healthy normal development.

Fig. 16. UNICEF conceptual framework for determinants of nutritional status

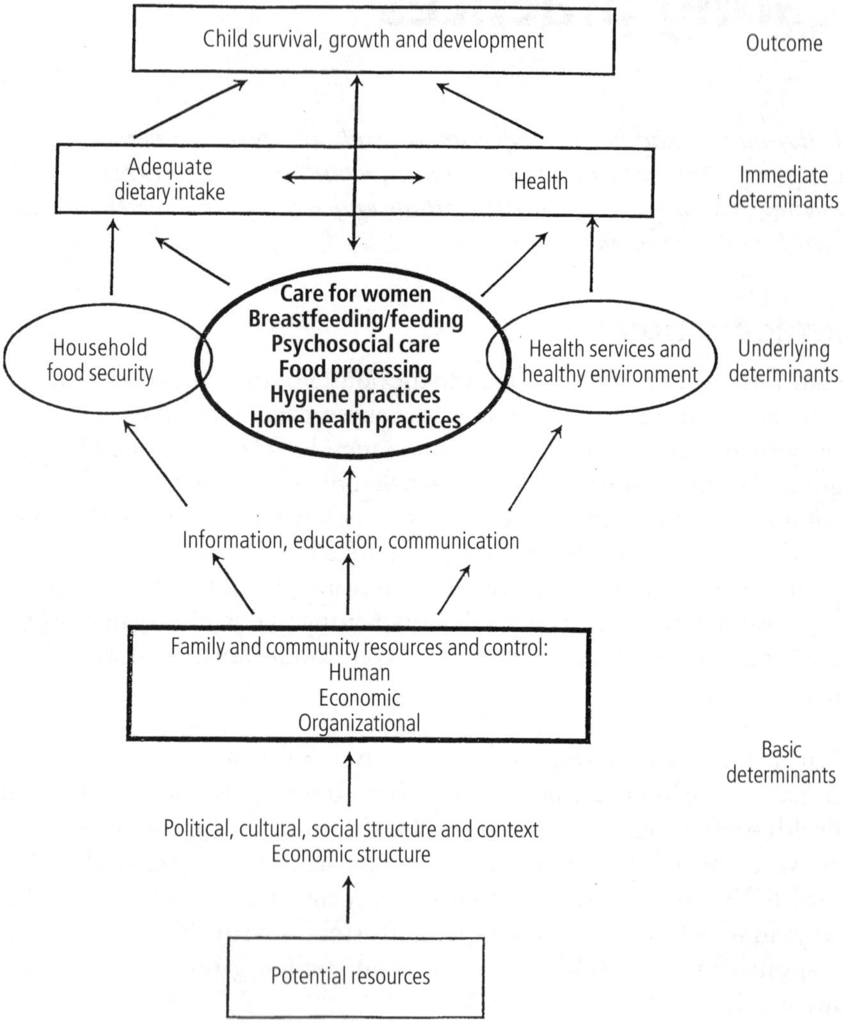

```
┌─────────────────────────────────────────────┐
│   Child survival, growth and development     │     Outcome
└─────────────────────────────────────────────┘

┌──────────────┐                    ┌──────────────┐
│  Adequate    │  ←──────────→      │   Health     │     Immediate
│ dietary intake│                    │              │     determinants
└──────────────┘                    └──────────────┘

            Care for women
         Breastfeeding/feeding
  Household  Psychosocial care   Health services and   Underlying
  food security  Food processing   healthy environment   determinants
         Hygiene practices
        Home health practices

       Information, education, communication

┌─────────────────────────────────────────────┐
│  Family and community resources and control: │
│                 Human                        │
│                Economic                      │
│              Organizational                  │
└─────────────────────────────────────────────┘
                                                      Basic
                                                      determinants

     Political, cultural, social structure and context
                  Economic structure

          ┌──────────────────────────┐
          │   Potential resources    │
          └──────────────────────────┘
```

Source: Engle et al. *(2)*.

A recent WHO review *(3)* demonstrates that nutrition interventions significantly improve both the psychological development and physical growth in poor and disadvantaged populations, and that combined psychosocial and nutrition interventions can have a greater impact than either alone. The premise behind interventions to promote growth and development simultaneously is that feeding behaviour that increases nutrient intake and psychological support for children's development require similar skills and resources from caregivers.

This chapter focuses on some important aspects of caring for children from conception to around 3 years of age, the most important period for child growth. For complementary feeding to be a success, not only must foods containing all necessary nutrients be available, but appropriate feeding behaviour is essential to ensure optimum development of the child. These types of behaviour, such as encouraging an anorexic child to eat or responding to a child's hunger, require that caregivers understand their significance and can act upon and implement them.

The UNICEF Care Initiative *(2)* and the WHO review *(3)* define the caring practices, the knowledge and the skills necessary to assess, analyse and take action to improve children's growth and development. Family practices necessary for good growth and development in children under the age of 3 years can be divided into the following six categories.

1. Care for women and girls includes: provision, by the household and/or community, of emotional and social support; ensuring food and rest during pregnancy and lactation; assessing workload; aiding recuperation from childbirth; promoting reproductive health; and respecting women's autonomy and decision-making.

2. Young child feeding includes: support for prompt initiation of exclusive, on-demand breastfeeding and its continuation for around the first 6 months of life (Chapter 7); protection from commercial pressures for formula feeding; the timely introduction of nutritionally adequate complementary foods (Chapter 8) with continued breastfeeding; and active as opposed to passive feeding.

3. Psychosocial care includes: responsive interaction with children and support for their development, including the acquisition of language and other communication skills through attention, affection and involvement; encouragement of exploration and learning; responsiveness to developmental milestones and cues; and protection from child abuse and violence.

4. Food preparation and related practices include: correct food storage and hygiene (Chapter 12).

5. Personal hygiene and household hygiene practices (Chapter 12) include: hand washing by the caregiver; bathing the child; having a clean house and play areas; using clean water and good sanitation; and protecting children from injury.

6. Home health practices involve: the care of children during illness, including the diagnosis of illness and timely referral to the health care
   services; prevention of illness through home-based protection measures
   such as use of oral rehydration solutions and control of mosquitos, rats
   and other pests; and the appropriate utilization of the health services.

These caring practices require resources and support from the family. Caring practices and resources vary greatly between cultures, and even within
different groups within cultures. However, children's basic need for food,
health care, protection, shelter and love are the same in all cultures. Widespread changes in society, such as urbanization and the changing economic
role of women, require adaptations in caring practices. Understanding the
importance of caring practices should help to identify good practices that
should be encouraged, and poor practices that need to be improved. Second, it will highlight the significance of strengthening families to be able to
provide the resources for these caring practices.

FACTORS AFFECTING THE ABILITY OF CAREGIVERS TO CARRY OUT OPTIMUM FEEDING PRACTICES

Research suggests that in almost all societies, mothers are the primary pro-
viders of care. Nevertheless, the amount of time a woman spends in direct
child care may decline rapidly as a child progresses from breastfeeding to
complementary feeding and becomes mobile. Furthermore, the mother's
employment often reduces the time available for child care. Fathers, other
relatives and institutions such as child care centres also provide care for
young children. In some cultures, siblings may be major caregivers.

Caregivers are constrained in their ability to provide the best care by a
number of factors. These can be divided into three main areas. First, education, knowledge and beliefs represent the capacity of the caregiver to provide appropriate care. Second, factors such as workload and time constraints, nutritional status, physical and mental health, stress and confidence all affect the caregiver's ability to turn his or her capacities into
behaviour and to implement them. Third, there are factors such as economic resources (including the caregiver's control of those resources) and
social support that facilitate this implementation. When caregivers are other
children, they want and need time to play and attend to their own activities,
which may be hindered by excessive caregiving. At the national level, resources
for care are influenced by social service expenditure priorities and poverty levels.
Political, cultural, social and economic structures constitute basic determinants
of the use of resources in support of families and caregivers for children.

CARE FOR GIRLS AND WOMEN AND THE CONSEQUENCES

The health and nutritional status of mothers before and during pregnancy and while lactating are crucial for the outcome of pregnancy and subsequently for normal child growth and development. Family support during this period will have a positive effect on birth outcomes. The care of women can be considered under several headings (Box 5).

Box 5. The care of women

During pregnancy and lactation
Provision of food
Workload and support
Facilitation of prenatal care and safe childbirth
Postpartum rest

Reproductive health
Delayed age at first pregnancy
Support for birth spacing

Physical health and nutritional status
Provision of food
Protection from physical abuse

Mental health, stress and self-confidence
Reduction of stress
Enhanced self-confidence and esteem
Protection from emotional abuse
Supportive social relations and companionship

Autonomy and respect within the family
Adequate decision-making power
Access to family income, assets and credit

Workload and time
Shared workload
Time for their families and themselves

Education
Support of equal access to education
Support of women's access to information

Source: Engle et al *(2)*.

A good quality diet during pregnancy and lactation is important for both mother and baby. This helps to reduce the risk of miscarriage, stillbirth and maternal mortality and helps to ensure an optimal micronutrient status for the infant (Chapter 7). Families can care for women by making sure that they receive the right amount of nutritious foods, including vegetables and fruit and a fair share of the family diet.

Anaemia and stunting in women are common in some countries of the Region, especially within vulnerable groups such as ethnic minorities and low-income families (see Chapter 6). These conditions are associated with increased maternal mortality and illness and with a high prevalence of low-birth-weight infants *(4,5)*. Child growth appears to be most affected during the prenatal period and the first 3 years of life. To encourage normal growth and to help prevent stunting, it is therefore important to ensure optimum nutritional status of pregnant women and of girls, particularly during the first years of life. Good nutritional status is important not only for a woman's reproductive role, but also for her productive role.

The breastfeeding component of good infant care can only be achieved when adequate attention is given to the care of the mother. Women who wish to practise exclusive breastfeeding (Chapter 7) and to continue breastfeeding during the complementary feeding period need information and counselling, and barriers to the initiation and continuation of breastfeeding should be removed. Fathers have been found to have a particularly important role in providing this support and in helping to remove potential barriers *(6)*.

The countries that emerged following the dissolution of the Soviet Union have seen a decline in prenatal services. The use of abortion as a contraceptive method has continued or even increased, and births to teenage girls and single women have risen. Studies suggest that knowledge of contraception and sexual health is limited. Delaying the age at which women begin childbearing until they have stopped growing will help to reduce risks for both mothers and their babies. Furthermore, increasing the space between successive births confers benefits to the mother, allowing maternal nutrient stores to be replenished and thereby reducing infant mortality and malnutrition. It is also vital to protect women from physical and emotional abuse, which affects their mental as well as their physical health.

FEEDING YOUNG CHILDREN

Sustained breastfeeding for 24 months or more is a crucial caring practice of the mother. Any form of infant feeding, other than exclusive breastfeeding, requires someone to spend time preparing food, ensuring hygiene during its preparation and storage, and feeding the food to the infant. Good hygiene practices are often compromised to save time.

Bottle feeding has many negative effects, especially in relation to hygiene. The bottle may be placed on the pillow beside the infant to save the caregiver's time. This deprives the infant of body and eye contact and psychosocial care. Unfortunately, families are often unaware of these risks and are poorly informed by health professionals.

Complementary foods are often introduced too early because it is thought that this will stop the infant crying so much, thus allowing the mother to get on with her work. Other efforts to save time include offering older infants gruels, either in self-feeding cups or in bottles (with the teat cut open to allow thicker fluid to pass through). Pacifiers are used for similar reasons. None of these practices is recommended. Any substitution for breast-milk in the first 6 months may result in a decline in the mother's milk supply; instead, the supply should be increased. Also, crying is often as much a signal of a need for care and comfort as one of hunger.

Active complementary feeding practice

The way in which caregivers facilitate feeding and encourage eating plays a major role in the food intake of infants and young children. There are four dimensions of appropriate feeding:

- adaptation of the feeding method to the psychomotor abilities of the child (ability to hold a spoon, ability to chew);

- responsiveness of the caregiver, including encouragement to eat, by offering additional foods;

- interaction with the caregiver, including the affective relationship; and

- the feeding situation, including the organization, frequency and regularity of feeding, and whether the child is supervised and protected while eating and by whom.

Adapting to the child's changing motor skills requires close attention by the caregiver, since these change rapidly during the first 2 years of life. The time required for a child to eat a specific amount decreases with age for solid and viscous foods, but not for thinner purées. Children's abilities to hold a spoon, handle a cup or grasp a piece of solid food also increase with age.

Caregivers need to be sure that children are capable of the self-feeding expected of them. Children also have a drive for independence, and may eat more if they are allowed to use newly learned finger skills to pick up foods.

Feeding responsively can be particularly important for young children. Caregivers can encourage, cajole, offer more helpings, talk to children while eating and monitor how much they eat. The amount of food that children consume may depend more on the caregiver's active encouragement than on the amount offered. Recommending that mothers encourage their children to eat may be as effective as telling mothers what to feed their children.

Caregivers who act as role models on how to eat healthily will encourage good eating habits in children. A relaxed and comfortable atmosphere without conflict will also facilitate good eating practices. With gentle encouragement and responsive feeding, evidence shows that children will often eat more than if they are left to eat on their own.

The caregiver's understanding of and response to cues of hunger in the child may be critical for the development of good feeding practices. For example, if caregivers interpret a child's mouth actions as refusal of a new food, they may stop feeding and so the child will receive less food.

Caregivers may not be aware of how much their children eat; one project found that when mothers paid more attention to the quantity of food their children ate, they were surprised by the small amounts and were willing to increase the amounts fed. Having a separate bowl for each child can help determine quantities eaten and encourage the slow eater. Often children will refuse food if the preferred caregiver is not present. Patience and understanding, together with recognition of the child's need to gain familiarity with the caregiver, will increase the chances of successful feeding.

There is a cultural spectrum of control with regard to eating. At one extreme the caregiver has all of the control, whereas at the other extreme control is given entirely to the child. Neither extreme is good for children. Too much control in the hands of the caregiver can result in force-feeding, or continued and even intrusive pressure on children to eat (7,8). Rather than providing an opportunity for interaction and cognitive and social enhancement, feeding can become a time of conflict resulting in the child refusing food. A responsive caregiver who can adapt to a child's refusals with gentle encouragement can often improve food intake.

At the other end of the spectrum, caregivers are passive and leave the initiative to eat to the child. At a certain age, children need and want autonomy in eating; before that time, however, too much autonomy will result in their not eating enough. Passive feeding may be due to lack of time and energy, or to a belief that children should not be pressured to eat. Although this belief may seem reasonable, extra encouragement may be necessary if a child has anorexia or a poor appetite. Caregivers have been observed to encourage feeding only after seeing that the child is refusing to eat, which may simply result in fruitless battles.

The environment in which children are fed may also influence their food intake. Children can be fed regularly each day, sitting in a set place where the food is easily accessible, or at the time that the caregiver finds most convenient. If the main meal is prepared late at night, children may fall asleep before it is completed. Children can be easily distracted, particularly if food is difficult to eat (such as soup with a spoon that the child is unable to use) or is not particularly tasty. If the supervision of feeding is not adequate, siblings or even animals may take advantage of a young child's vulnerability and take food away, or food may be spilled on the ground. The best feeding situation for a child is a familiar place protected from distractions and intrusions.

Adaptation to the family diet
The transition from breastfeeding and transitional foods to the normal family diet and cessation of breastfeeding should be gradual, allowing the child to return to the breast occasionally. By the second year, unadapted family foods are an appropriate complement to breastfeeding as the child takes increasing quantities of food (Chapter 8). Caregivers may expect children to feed themselves during this transition. If these expectations are too great, the child may not get enough food. Caregivers should continue to be aware of how much the child is eating, and of the possibility of anorexia.

Many studies have documented the importance of the relationship between the caregiver and the child, and the organization of the eating situation in relation to poor child growth. A number of characteristics differentiate feeding situations in which children fail to thrive with those in which they grow normally. Factors associated with failure to thrive include: an authoritarian, disciplinary approach that may override the child's internal regulation of hunger; low maternal responsiveness and sensitivity to cues; a family atmosphere that is not supportive or cohesive; and possibly difficult personalities (9). Strategies that use behaviour modification to alter these relationships have resulted in positive changes in feeding practices (10). More research is needed into how feeding practices can best be modified, particularly in situations of nonresponsive feeding, including very passive feeding or force-feeding.

The response of the caregiver to the child's appetite can lead to the child demanding less food. When food is scarce, caregivers may tend to discourage children from requesting food, leading to a lower food intake when it becomes more plentiful. Sometimes caregivers feel that a child should learn not to ask for food, or that an immediate response to a child's request for food represents "spoiling" or inappropriate indulgence. In these cases, the chances of the child achieving adequate intake are reduced, since demand plays a significant role in the amount of food ingested. Snacks between meals are sometimes an important source of extra energy.

On the other hand, overfeeding and overweight in children are emerging as important public health problems in the European Region (see Chapter 10). Often diets are high in energy (from added fats and sugars) and low in micronutrients, and energy intakes are higher than necessary. Again, feeding practices and attitudes about feeding play a significant role in generating and preventing overnutrition.

PSYCHOSOCIAL CARE

The caregiver's attention, affection, and involvement, and encouragement of autonomy, exploration and learning (Box 6) are correlated with better nutritional status in the child.

Box 6. Psychosocial care of the young child

Responsiveness to developmental milestones and cues
Adapting interaction to child's developmental stage
Attention to low activity levels and slow development of the child

Attention, affection and involvement
Frequent positive interactions (touching, holding, talking)

Encouragement of autonomy, exploration and learning
Encouragement of playing, exploration, talking
Adoption of a teaching or guiding role

Prevention of and protection from abuse and violence

Source: Engle et al. (2).

The responsiveness of the caregiver to developmental milestones and cues affects the child's growth and development. This includes the extent to which caregivers are aware of children's signals and needs, interpret them accurately, and respond to them promptly, appropriately and consistently *(11)*.

The attention, affection and involvement that caregivers show to children influence their growth and development. The most important factor in a child's healthy development is to have at least one strong relationship with a caring adult who values the wellbeing of the child. Lack of a consistent caregiver can create additional risks for children.

RESOURCES FOR CARE

The resources needed to support caring practices are human resources, such as knowledge or health, and economic and organizational resources (Box 7) *(12)*. These resources have direct effects on caring practices, and therefore on child growth and development. They also have indirect effects, such as facilitating access to enough food, the use of health services and the healthiness of the environment in which a child grows and develops. Resources for care can be identified at family and community levels, and are influenced by political, social and economic structures and by the cultural context.

Box 7. Resources for care

Human resources
Education, knowledge and beliefs
Health and nutritional status of the caregiver
Mental health, stress and self-confidence
Fathers and men in families

Economic resources
Control of family resources and assets
Workload and time

Organizational resources
Alternative caregivers
Community support for care
Legislation for maternity leave
Mother and child welfare schemes

Source: Engle et al. *(2)*

Human resources

The risks to children arising from absence of human resources have risen dramatically in the former Soviet countries. Marriage rates have declined, divorce rates have increased, fertility has decreased, and a greater percentage of births are to teenage and single mothers. There has been an increase in families with only one parent, some 30% in the Russian Federation, for example *(13)*. Furthermore, a high number of deaths has been recorded, most commonly among middle-aged men. These changes reduce children's access to caregiving, and specifically to the resources provided by two parents *(13)*.

Smoking and alcohol use and abuse have increased over the past 10 years in the countries of central and eastern Europe. These habits have a negative impact both on caregivers – damaging their health and thereby reducing their ability to care – and on children through both prenatal and postnatal exposure. Alcohol abuse can reduce the effectiveness of both mothers and fathers and is thought to be a major factor contributing to the excess mortality in the Region.

A caregiver's good health can improve the care of children. When caregivers are ill, they are less able to provide optimal care for children. Very little research exists on the associations between the nutritional status of the mother, in particular that of iron, and caregiving. The lower activity levels of anaemic compared to nonanaemic women in an Egyptian study suggest that women with anaemia have less energy to devote to child care. Anaemia is also associated with fatigue, apathy and loss of mental concentration, all of which can undermine a caregiver's ability to look after children *(14)*.

It should not be forgotten that some teenage mothers have not completed their growth and attained their adult weight and height. Their nutritional needs may be as important as, and compete with, those of their infants.

There is a large body of literature demonstrating a positive association between the educational level of caregivers and their children's health and nutritional status *(15)*. More educated mothers tend to have greater knowledge of nutrition *(16)*, greater assertiveness and higher status within the household, better ability to make use of health care systems, and greater capacity to allocate resources on their own. They may also have more hygienic household practices and personal habits and a greater knowledge of appropriate child rearing. Thus, education of caregivers is one of the most important investments that can be made in children's growth and development. It is vital to assess current knowledge and beliefs, in order to identify existing practices that should be supported.

Research in the United States *(11)* has shown links between the quality of psychosocial care a child receives and his or her growth and nutritional status. A caregiver with depression or anxiety, who is living under considerable stress, or who lacks support and control over resources will find it difficult to provide patient, loving care. Evidence from industrialized countries suggests that depressed women are less able to provide adequate care for their children, with long-term emotional and behavioural consequences for the children.

In large families with many children, infants may be at risk of neglect. This has certainly been demonstrated in developing countries, where the "weaned" child (lately displaced from the breast) is at particular nutritional risk. In developed countries, failure to thrive is much more common in children of poorer families where there is – in addition to poor infant diet and feeding practices – inadequate parenting (including parental psychopathology, poor parent–child interaction and family dysfunction *(17–19)*).

Fathers represent an important human resource for the care of their children. In many cultures, however, fathers may be restricted by cultural and personal attitudes from greater roles in child care, despite often having more free time than mothers. Fathers can have a positive effect on caregiving by supporting mothers in breastfeeding and obtaining health care, sharing more of the workload, and providing direct child care.

Economic resources

In many parts of the WHO European Region, increasing poverty levels and the widening gap between the wealthy and the poor have led to a significant deterioration in household incomes. Real wages and employment rates have dropped in many countries, resulting in greater disparity in income. Rising poverty levels result in families using a higher proportion of their household budget on food and consuming less energy, and the emergence of new risk factors such as poverty-related diseases and drug abuse *(13)*.

The poverty level of a family is one of the most important risk factors for poor child health and nutrition. Nevertheless, the child's nutritional status can be determined by the person in the household making decisions on resource allocation. Evidence suggests that mothers are more likely than fathers to allocate resources to children, and that the greater the proportion of the household income earned by women the more likely the child will benefit in terms of health and nutrition *(20–22)*. Studies also suggest that children living in households headed by women or with single mothers sometimes do better than would be expected from the family income.

The time that women have to spend on other activities, including earning an income, food production and preparation and household duties, are important constraints on child care. In the absence of other adequate caregivers or support from the family and community, the increased income from working may not offset the loss of time available for child care.

The impact of women's employment on children's nutritional status and health outcomes is not clear-cut. Perhaps more important than work *per se* is the availability of a substitute caregiver, such as an adult female relative, who can provide high-quality care in the absence of the mother. Wage rates have also been found to affect children's welfare. Where mothers are involved in formal work or have a reasonable income, and have adequate alternative caregivers, there appears to be no negative impact on the child's nutritional status *(20,23)*. Nevertheless, the children of women who are poorly paid, or who work long hours for little pay, have a relatively poor nutritional status *(24,25)*.

The value of investing time in child care and stimulation of child development is not always obvious to parents. Unless parents perceive that additional time with children will have some benefit to themselves or to their children, strategies to increase their available time will probably have only minimal effects on time devoted to child care *(11)*.

Organizational resources

Owing to changes in society, fewer adults are available to provide supervision for their children, and there are fewer community organizations to provide support in many parts of the Region. In some countries in eastern Europe there has been an increase in the number of children in public care, such as "infant homes", orphanages, boarding schools and institutions for children with disabilities *(13)*. The majority of these children in public care are "social orphans", children who cannot be cared for by their families because of abandonment, parental death, illness or imprisonment, or harmful or neglectful parenting. Despite hopes that, following the dissolution of the Soviet Union, large numbers of these children would be placed with families, the percentage of children in public care has increased in most of the countries for which there are data *(13)*.

The support that the primary caregiver receives can include child care assistance, information or emotional support. Alternative child care is one of the most important types of social support, and the abilities of another caregiver to provide care has particular relevance to complementary feeding. Different degrees of care are needed at the different stages of child development. In the first year of life, care provided by anyone other than the mother or a competent caregiver is associated with higher infant morbidity and possibly mortality. Care needs remain high in the second year of life, although the shortcomings of the caregiver can be ameliorated to some extent if good quality food is available and the environment is both healthy and safe. By the third year of life, many children are becoming less dependent.

Poor families, mothers in difficult situations, sickly or disabled children, and marginalized and uneducated parents need support and are the least likely to get it. They may not be able to seek help because they lack contacts, do not know where to go and feel looked down upon. The community needs to be made aware of the greater vulnerability of and the risks faced by some caregivers and children.

Community support for caregiving is an important resource for families. For example, the Baby Friendly Hospital Initiative and other efforts that improve the sensitivity and skills of health workers to infant feeding and care provide valuable support for families from the start. After this, informal support from family and neighbours, community care services, day care facilities, and parenting education and activities are all essential. Health care systems based in communities can reduce the time that women spend in obtaining care, and can improve the responsiveness of the health care system to the needs of the child in the community.

The state's policies on employment, prices, incomes, subsidies, health, education and agriculture, and the legal system, can influence resources for care. Legal actions, such as ratifying the Convention on the Rights of the Child, can improve care. In many countries, however, enforceable legislation to support these initiatives is lacking. Political support for caregiving should include legislation to protect the entitlement of women to maternity leave and nursing breaks, as recommended in the Innocenti Declaration *(26,27*; and see Annex 1, page *272)*. Without maternity leave the poorer the woman, the sooner she will have to return to work. Discrimination against women in the workplace, or unequal opportunities for women, should be avoided in order to improve care. Ratification of the International Code of Marketing of Breast-milk Substitutes and subsequent relevant resolutions of the World Health Assembly (see Chapter 7 and Annex 1) will also improve care.

Some countries provide direct support to women and infants. In the United Kingdom the Welfare Food Scheme, originally designed (in 1948) as a universal programme regardless of income, currently benefits around 25%

of 0–4-year-olds living in households that receive income support. The scheme provides free milk and vitamin supplements to pregnant and lactating women and their children and milk formula to infants. The scheme also provides for disabled children and those who attend day-care facilities. The value of the scheme in terms of its effects on the nutritional status of the infants has not been formally evaluated, but it is widely regarded as providing an important "safety net" for potentially vulnerable children of low-income families. The Department of Health commissioned a scientific review of the Welfare Food Scheme in 2000 *(28)*.

In the United States, the Special Supplemental Nutrition Program for Women, Infants and Children (WIC) also aims to improve the nutritional status and health of low-income families by providing food supplements, nutrition education and coordinated health care to pregnant, breastfeeding and postpartum women and preschool children. The WIC Program provides:

- infants up to 12 months with iron-fortified infant formula (if not breastfed);
- infants aged 6–12 months with iron-fortified cereal and vitamin C-fortified juice;
- children aged 1–5 years with milk, iron-fortified cereal, eggs, vitamin C or citrus juice, cheese and dried beans; and
- breastfeeding women with milk, cheese, iron-fortified cereal, eggs, vitamin C or citrus juice and dried beans.

A number of studies have described the benefits of the WIC Program. In addition to reducing the number of low-birth-weight babies *(29)*, infant growth (between 6 and 18 months) has been improved *(30)* and childhood iron deficiency anaemia has been reduced, particularly among low-income families *(31)*.

REFERENCES

1. *World Declaration and Plan of Action for Nutrition.* Geneva, World Health Organization, 1992 (document ICN/92/2).
2. ENGLE, P.L. ET AL. *The Care Initiative. Assessment, analysis and action to improve care for nutrition.* New York, United Nations Children's Fund, 1997.
3. *A critical link: interventions for physical growth and psychological development.* Geneva, World Health Organization, 1999 (document WHO/CHS/CAH/99.3).

4. MARTORELL, R. ET AL. Reproductive performance and nutrition during childhood. *Nutrition reviews*, **54**: S15–S21 (1996).

5. LESLIE, J. Improving the nutrition of women in the third world. *In*: Pinstrup-Andersen, P. et al., ed. *Child growth and nutrition in developing countries. Priorities for action.* Ithaca, NY, Cornell University Press, 1994, pp. 117–138.

6. GREINER, T. Sustained breastfeeding, complementation and care. *Food and nutrition bulletin*, **16**: 313–319 (1995).

7. BROWN, K.H. ET AL. Consumption of weaning foods from fermented cereals: Kwara State, Nigeria. *In*: Alnwick, D. et al., ed. *Improving young child feeding in Eastern and Southern Africa household-level food technology. Proceedings of a workshop held in Nairobi, Kenya, 12 October 1987.* Ottawa, International Development Research Council, 1988, pp. 181–197.

8. DETTWYLER, K.A. Interaction of anorexia and cultural beliefs in infant malnutrition in Mali. *American journal of human biology*, **1**: 683–695 (1989).

9. BLACK, M. Failure to thrive: strategies for evaluation and intervention. *School psychology review*, **24**: 171–185 (1995).

10. LARSON, K.L. ET AL. A behavioral feeding program for failure-to-thrive infants. *Behaviour research and therapy*, **25**: 39–47 (1987).

11. ENGLE, P.L. & RICCIUTI, H.N. Psychosocial aspects of care and nutrition. *Food and nutrition bulletin*, **16**: 356–377 (1995).

12. JONSSON, U. Ethics and child nutrition. *Food and nutrition bulletin*, **16**: 293–298 (1995).

13. *Children at risk in central and eastern Europe: perils and promises.* Florence, UNICEF International Child Development Centre, 1997 (Regional Monitoring Report, No.4).

14. WINKVIST, A. Health and nutritional status of the caregiver: effect on caregiving capacity. *Food and nutrition bulletin*, **16**: 389–397 (1995).

15. *Complementary feeding of young children in developing countries: a review of current scientific knowledge.* Geneva, World Health Organization, 1998 (document WHO/NUT/98.1).

16. RUEL, M.T. ET AL. The mediating effect of maternal nutrition knowledge on the association between maternal schooling and child nutritional status in Lesotho. *American journal of epidemiology*, **135**: 904–914 (1992).

17. SKUSE, D. ET AL. Psychosocial adversity and growth during infancy. *European journal of clinical nutrition*, **48**: 113–130 (1994).

18. WRIGHT, C. ET AL. Effect of deprivation on weight gain in infancy. *Acta paediatrica*, **83**: 357–359 (1994).

19. RAYNOR, P. & RUDLOF, M. What do we know about children who fail to thrive? *Child care, health and development*, **22**: 241–250 (1996).

20. ENGLE, P.L. Maternal work and child care strategies in peri-urban Guatemala: nutritional effects. *Child development*, **62**: 954–965 (1991).
21. ENGLE, P.L. Influences of mothers' and fathers' income on child nutritional status in Guatemala. *Social science and medicine*, **37**: 1303–1312 (1993).
22. JOHNSON, F.C. & ROGERS, B.L. Children's nutritional status in female-based households in the Dominican Republic. *Social science and medicine*, **37**: 1293–1301 (1993).
23. VIAL, I. & MUCHNIK, E. Women, market work, infant feeding and infant nutrition among low-income women in Santiago, Chile. *In*: Leslie, J. & Paolisso, M., ed. *Women, work, and child welfare in the Third World*. Boulder, CO, West View Publishing, 1989.
24. LAMONTAGNE, J. ET AL. Maternal employment and nutritional status of 12–18 month old children in Managua, Nicaragua. *Social science and medicine*, **46**: 403–414 (1998).
25. POWELL, C.A. & GRANTHAM MCGREGOR, S. The ecology of nutritional status and development in young children in Kingston, Jamaica. *American journal of clinical nutrition*, **41**: 1322–1331 (1985).
26. *International Labour Conference, 87th Session. Report V (1): maternity protection at work. Revisions of the Maternity Protection Convention (revised), 1952 (No. 103), and Recommendation, 1952 (No. 95)*. Geneva, International Labour Organization, 1999.
27. *Comparative analysis of implementation of the Innocenti Declaration in WHO European Member States. Monitoring Innocenti targets on the protection, promotion and support of breastfeeding*. Copenhagen, WHO Regional Office for Europe, 1999 (document EUR/ICP/LVNG 01 01 02).
28. DEPARTMENT OF HEALTH, UNITED KINGDOM. *UK review of Welfare Food Scheme*. London, Stationery Office, 2000 (in press).
29. BROWN, H.C. ET AL. The impact of the WIC food supplement program on birth outcomes. *American journal of obstetrics and gynecology*, **174**: 1279–1283 (1996).
30. HEIMENDINGER, J. ET AL. The effects of the WIC program on the growth of infants. *American journal of clinical nutrition*, **40**: 1250–1257 (1984).
31. MILLER, C. ET AL. Impact of WIC Program on the iron status of infants. *Pediatrics*, **75**: 100–105 (1985).

CHAPTER 10

Growth assessment

Regular growth monitoring is an important tool for assessing the nutritional status of infants and young children and should be an integral part of the child health care system.

INTRODUCTION

During the first 6 months of life, infants grow faster than at any other time after birth, gaining about 200 g and almost 1 cm per week. Full-term infants triple their weight and increase their length by 50% during the first year. In late infancy, although growth rate slows down, it remains high compared to that in childhood (Table 45). Because of this rapid growth rate nutritional requirements per kilogram of body weight are very high, and the amount of protein and energy required for growth is a critical component of the total needs (see Chapter 3).

Infants and young children are very vulnerable to growth faltering as a result of malnutrition. In populations where nutritional problems are present, it is common for both weight and height to deviate progressively from the growth reference *(1)* during the period of complementary feeding when the quality and quantity of the diet are inadequate.

There are also indications that the secular trend of increasing adult stature, which has been seen in many European countries over the last decades *(2)*, is

Table 45. Average expected gain in weight, length and head circumference during the first 2 years of life					
	Age				
	0–3 months	3–6 months	6–9 months	9–12 months	12–24 months
Average expected weight gain (kg)	2.5	1.8	1.4	0.9	2.5
Average expected length gain (cm)	10	7	5	4	10
Average expected gain in head circumference (cm)	5.4	3.0	1.8	1.4	2.2

primarily due to improved growth performance in the first years of life and it is likely that nutrition plays a strong role in this process. This reduction of stunting in early life has been associated with increased social and economic development in developing countries (3).

HOW TO MEASURE GROWTH AND USE GROWTH CHARTS

Growth is an increase in the mass and dimensions of the body and comprises weight (ponderal) and length or height (linear) components. The accurate measurement of both components is essential when assessing growth. Standardization of technique and calibration of equipment are essential to ensure accurate and reliable measurements. Digital (electronic) scales should be used whenever possible, and the child should be lightly clothed and without shoes when weighed. Length (rather than height) is generally measured up to 2 years of age (second birthday) and height thereafter. The former is measured using a length board or mat and the latter with a stadiometer. The United Nations' *Reference on practical measurements in children (4)* is a useful guide to carrying out these measurements.

To obtain meaningful information about infant and child growth, several consecutive measurements should be obtained, including birth data, and plotted on growth charts derived from appropriate reference populations. It is recommended that weight, length (height) and head circumference be measured at birth and regularly during infancy and childhood, for instance monthly for the first 3 months, every 3 months until 1 year, and thereafter every 6 months.

Fig. 17 gives examples of growth charts of weight-for-age, length-for-age and weight-for-length for boys covering the 3 first years of life. The charts are constructed from data from the current WHO reference (5). Each chart has three curves: the median or 50th percentile and the 3rd and 97th percentiles. The 3rd and 97th percentiles are approximately equivalent to the –2 SD and +2 SD curves, respectively. Charts for boys and girls are different and can be colour-coded for convenience.

When a child is measured, the value should be plotted on the chart as a dot. If the measurement is, for example, on the 25th percentile curve it means that, compared with the reference population, 25% of the children have a value below this and 75% a value above. If the measurement is either below the 3rd percentile or above the 97th percentile the value is regarded as "abnormal".

Measurements at one point in time, without reference to earlier recordings, make it impossible to determine whether the child is following steadily along a growth percentile, moving downwards or catching up. Deficits in different indices reflect different underlying processes and suggest different causations. Weight can be lost and gained quickly in response to environmental insults, while height cannot be lost. Wasting and stunting are terms coined to reflect these different processes (see below).

Because single anthropometric measurements (such as height or weight) are of limited value, derived indices (such as weight-for-height, length-for-age and weight-for-length) should instead be calculated. These allow growth data to be compared within and between groups, and take into account the sex of the child.

REFERENCE POPULATIONS

Three indices of attained growth can be calculated by comparing an individual child to a reference population: weight-for-age, height-for-age and weight-for-height. The body mass index (weight/height^2) has also been recommended in children, but it is not widely used before the age of 10 years (6).

The value of a growth index is that it shows the position of an individual child in relation to the distribution of weights (or heights) of children of equal age and sex. Growth indices can be expressed in one of three ways:

- as a deviation from the median of the reference expressed as a standard deviation (SD or Z score);

- as a centile of the reference population; or

- as a percentage of the median reference value.

For the analysis of data, SD or Z scores are recommended because they lend themselves to easy mathematical manipulation and statistical analysis (7,8).

WHO has endorsed the use of populations defined by the US National Center for Health Statistics (NCHS) as a reference (6). However, the use of references based on a population of infants and children from one country to assess the growth of children in another country has proved controversial. Differences in the genetic potential for growth are often quoted as a rationale for having country- or region-specific growth references.

Fig. 17. Examples of growth charts based on the WHO reference for boys for the first 3 years

A. Weight-for-age

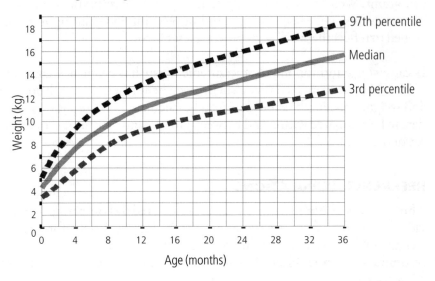

B. Length-for-age

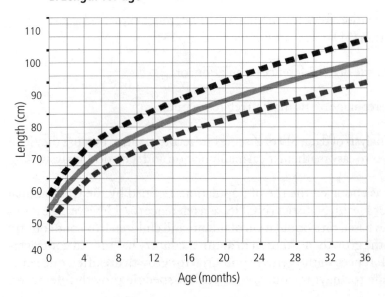

Fig. 17 (contd)

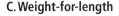

C. Weight-for-length

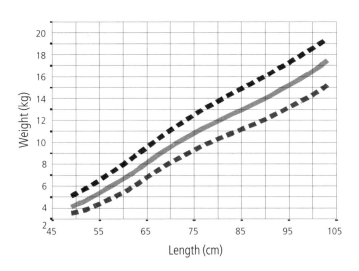

Length (cm)

Source: World Health Organization *(5)*.

Nevertheless, while genetic differences exist, it is environmental factors that have the larger effect on the potential for growth. Martorell, who measured the heights of school-age children from different socioeconomic groups in different countries, demonstrated this clearly *(9)*.

WHO has acknowledged that reference data will be used as standards, and recommends that care be taken to choose references that resemble international standards *(6)*. WHO chose the NCHS reference because the population on which it was based lived in a healthy environment, was well nourished and had probably met its full growth potential. As a standard, however, its limitations must be recognized. The growth curves were originally constructed in 1975 from four sources. The 0–23-month data of recumbent lengths came from the Fels Research Institute Longitudinal Study of 1923–1975. The infants included in this data set were predominately formula-fed (that is, not exclusively breastfed) and were from a relatively restricted genetic, socioeconomic and geographical background. The 2–18-year-old data of standing heights came from three American surveys between 1960 and 1975. Across most populations there is little difference in mean growth in height or in the distribution around the mean, but the inclusion of both healthy and sick, breast-fed and formula-fed infants in this reference should be remembered, particularly when comparing individuals or particular groups against the reference. A WHO Expert Committee (6) has recently recommended the development of a new growth reference for infants and children based on groups of infants breastfed according to WHO recommendations from different parts of the world.

INTERPRETATION OF MEASUREMENTS OF ATTAINED GROWTH

One of the major uses of derived growth indices is to predict subsequent health problems, especially morbidity, mortality, intellectual development, work capacity, reproductive performance and risk of chronic disease. However, prediction does not necessarily indicate causation. There was a strong exponential association between weight-for-age and mortality rates in a meta-analysis of six longitudinal studies of children, but its capacity to predict death was low (10). Its predictive value was highest in populations with high morbidity and mortality, indicating that malnutrition increases case fatality rates rather than the incidence of disease.

Weight-for-length is a better index of acute risk than weight-for-age and therefore of more value in identifying children who need nutritional treatment (11). The choice of a cut-off point for an index of attained growth is required to define the indicators needed for public health and policy decisions. Cut-off points are selected on operational grounds (for example, how many beneficiaries an aid programme can afford) or, more appropriately, on the basis of the risk of morbidity and mortality associated to a certain level of the indices. It has been shown, however, that the relationship between the indices and risk is continuous, but differs between countries according to the compounded environmental risk (10).

A cut-off of < 70% of reference median is commonly used as an indicator in developing countries for admission to hospital with severe malnutrition. UNICEF defines children as being moderately/severely underweight, wasted or stunted as those with < 2 SD compared with the reference (NCHS) median weight-for-age, weight-for-height and height-for-age, respectively. Using these definitions, 30% (170 million) and 40% (230 million) of the world's children are moderately/severely underweight or stunted, respectively. The prevalence of low weight-for-height (wasting) and that of low height-for-age (stunting), as defined above, are considered the main indicators of infant nutrition in a country.

Weight-for-height
A low weight-for-height results either from a failure to gain weight or from weight loss. It can develop rapidly, be reversed rapidly and is an index of acute undernutrition reflecting severe weight loss, which is often associated with acute starvation and/or severe illness. Wasting is not prevalent in the WHO European Region except in Tajikistan and Uzbekistan (see Chapter 1).

Studies from the early 1970s suggested that excessive weight-for-length (fatness) during infancy could result in a lifelong risk of obesity. More recent epidemiological studies, however, show no strong correlation between fatness during infancy and obesity in later life (12,13) and fatness during infancy may even have positive effects. Adult obesity and its cardiovascular consequences appear to have their origins during older childhood (14,15), but the degree to which fatness during early childhood (second and third years of life) is associated with obesity in later life is not known.

Height-for-age
A low height-for-age results from slowing of skeletal growth. In general it reflects a chronic process and is used as an index of chronic undernutrition. Stunting often develops within a fairly short period, from several months after birth to about 2 years of age. This coincides with the time when complementary foods are first introduced into the diet. Premature birth and intrauterine growth retardation are also the cause of an earlier onset of stunting, linked to impairment of glucose tolerance during adult life (16). Associated with the process of early nutritional stunting are: an elevated mortality risk; delayed motor development; impaired cognitive function and school performance; reduced lean body mass; and impaired work performance in adulthood with corresponding adverse economic consequences, suggesting that some of the factors causing stunting also have long-term adverse effects (3,17).

Impairment of linear growth is multifactorial. The most important causal factors are poor nutrition, infection (often caused by poor sanitary conditions) and poor mother–infant interaction and caregiver practices (see Chapter 9). Addressing the problems of malnutrition, treating infection and improving mother–infant interaction is recommended in a combined strategy, such as the Integrated Management of Childhood Illness (18), to prevent stunting in a resource-poor environment because this combined strategy will also improve physical and cognitive development.

Weight-for-age

Weight-for-age encompasses both weight-for-height and height-for-age. As an index of nutritional status it has limitations. A child with a low weight-for-age can be stunted and have a relatively normal weight-for-height. In younger children, low weight-for-age may reflect the prevalence of low weight-for-height, but in older age groups is more likely to be associated with a low height-for-age.

CATCH-UP GROWTH

Catch-up growth is possible after growth faltering, and requires reversal of nutrient deficiency *(19,20)*. Catch-up growth will only occur, however, if an appropriate diet is available over a sufficient period of time. It is still not clear which specific components of the diet are critical *(21)*. Generally, catch-up growth requires an increased amount of energy, protein and micronutrients, and these are in addition to the extra needs during the period of recovery from infection. Intervening may have only a limited effect although there is evidence that prolongation of the growth period, accelerated growth rates and improvement in the environment have positive effects on catch-up growth *(22)*.

REFERENCES

1. WEAVER, L.T. Feeding the weanling in the developing world: problems and solutions. *International journal of food sciences and nutrition*, **45**: 127–134 (1994).
2. SCHMIDT, I.M. ET AL. Height of conscripts in Europe – is postneonatal mortality a predictor? *Annals of human biology*, **22**: 57–67 (1995).
3. MARTORELL, R. The nature of child malnutrition and its long term implications. *Food and nutrition bulletin*, **20**: 288–292 (1999).
4. *Reference on practical measurements in children: National Household Survey Capability Programme. How to weigh and measure children.* New York, United Nations, 1986 (DP/UN/INT-81-041/6E).
5. *Measuring change in nutritional status.* Geneva, World Health Organization, 1983.
6. *Physical status: the use and interpretation of anthropometry.* Geneva, World Health Organization, 1995 (WHO Technical Report Series, No. 854).
7. WATERLOW, J.C. ET AL. The presentation and use of height and weight data for comparing nutritional status of groups of children under the age of 10 years. *Bulletin of the World Health Organization*, **55**: 489–498 (1977).

8. Use and interpretation of anthropometric indicators of nutritional status. *Bulletin of the World Health Organization*, 64: 929–941 (1986).

9. MARTORELL, R. Child growth retardation: a discussion of its causes and of its relationship to health. *In*: Blaxter, K.L. & Waterlow, J.C., ed. *Nutritional adaptation in man.* London, John Libbey, 1985, pp. 13–30.

10. PELLETIER, D.L. ET AL. Epidemiologic evidence for a potentiating effect of malnutrition on child mortality. *American journal of public health*, 83: 1130–1133 (1993).

11. BERN, C. ET AL. Assessment of potential indicators for protein–energy malnutrition in the algorithm for integrated management of childhood illness. *Bulletin of the World Health Organization*, 75 (Suppl. 1): 87–96 (1997).

12. ROLLAND-CACHERA, M.F. ET AL. Tracking the development of adiposity from one month of age to adulthood. *Annals of human biology*, 14: 219–229 (1987).

13. ROBERTS, S.B. Early diet and obesity. *In*: Heird, W.C., ed. *Nutritional needs of the six to twelve month old infant.* New York, Raven Press, 1991.

14. SINAIKO, A.R. ET AL. Relation of weight and rate of increase in weight during childhood and adolescence to body size, blood pressure, fasting insulin, and lipids in young adults. The Minneapolis Children's Blood Pressure Study. *Circulation,* 99: 1471–1476 (1999).

15. EPSTEIN, L.H. ET AL. Childhood obesity. *Pediatric clinics of North America,* 32: 363–379 (1985).

16. OZANNE, S.E. & HALES, C.N. The long-term consequences of intrauterine protein malnutrition for glucose metabolism. *Proceedings of the Nutrition Society,* 58: 615–619 (1999).

17. HERNANDEZ-DIAZ, S. ET AL. Association of maternal short stature with stunting in Mexican children: common genes vs common environment. *European journal of clinical nutrition*, 53: 938–945 (1999).

18. *A critical link: interventions for physical growth and psychological development.* Geneva, World Health Organization, 1999 (document WHO/CHS/CAH/99.3).

19. WATERLOW, J.C. Nutrition and growth. *In: Protein energy malnutrition.* London, Edward Arnold, 1985, pp. 187–211.

20. *Management of severe malnutrition: a manual for physicians and other senior health workers.* Geneva, World Health Organization, 1999.

21. GOLDEN, M.H.N. Is complete catch-up possible for stunted malnourished children? *European journal of clinical nutrition*, 48 (Suppl. 1): 58–68 (1994).

22. MARTORELL, R. ET AL. Reversibility of stunting: epidemiological findings in children from developing countries. *European journal of clinical nutrition*, 48 (Suppl. 1): 45–57 (1994).

CHAPTER II

Dental health

It is recommended that the frequent intake of foods high in sugar, sugary drinks, sweets and refined sugar should be limited to improve dental health.

Teeth should be cleaned gently twice a day as soon as they appear.

An optimal fluoride intake should be secured through water fluoridation, fluoride supplements or the use of fluoride toothpaste.

PREVALENCE OF DENTAL CARIES

Dental caries (tooth decay), a major health and social problem in many industrialized countries and in those in transition, is the most important dental problem in young children. Despite a decrease in prevalence over the last 20 years, this trend has reached a plateau, especially in preschool children, a considerable proportion of whom are still affected by dental caries. In the United Kingdom, for example, more than 50% of 5-year-old children suffer from tooth decay. Higher levels of caries are found in children from economically disadvantaged communities compared with those from more affluent areas, and dental caries is also more common in children of families that have recently immigrated. In the developing world the pattern is reversed, with affluent families tending to have adverse dietary habits that lead to a greater incidence of dental caries.

Within Europe, the countries of central and eastern Europe and those that emerged following the dissolution of the Soviet Union continue to suffer from high caries levels that significantly exceed those found in other European countries. These are well above the European average, and do not reach the WHO target for the year 2000 of a population average DMFT (decayed, missing and filled teeth) index of ≤ 3.0 *(1)*. Furthermore, unlike in most of western Europe, the distribution of the disease is not concentrated in certain groups but still affects the vast majority of people from an early age. Fig. 18 shows the prevalence of dental caries in Europe between 1982 and 1995.

Dental disease is not an inevitable part of life, and it can be greatly reduced by effective parent-targeted dental health education. Establishing good dental and eating habits in infancy and early childhood is central to long-term dental health.

Fig. 18. The prevalence of dental caries in Europe, 1982–1988 and 1989–1995

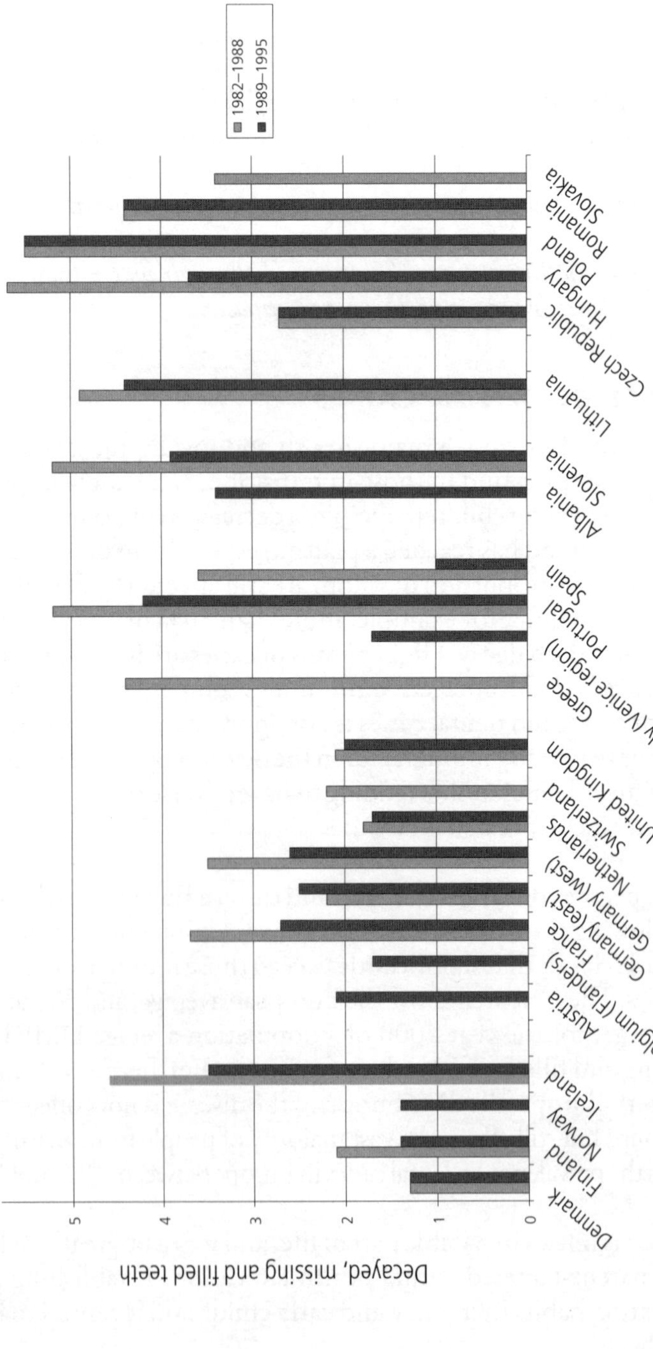

Source: adapted from Marthaler (1).

HOW CARIES ARE FORMED

The process of caries formation begins when the enamel at the tooth surface becomes demineralized (softened), with the loss of calcium and phosphate. The destruction spreads to the softer, sensitive, deeper part of the tooth, the dentine (beneath the enamel), and the weakened enamel then collapses to form a cavity. The process continues, progressively destroying the tooth.

Caries is caused by the action of organic acids on the tooth enamel. The acid is the by-product of the metabolism of dietary carbohydrates, primarily sugars, by the bacteria present in the layer of plaque covering tooth surfaces. Growth and extension of plaque is promoted by sugars, and a high-sugar diet encourages the multiplication of bacteria that use sugars as their source of energy and can efficiently convert them to acid. The plaque not only traps acid against the tooth surface but also acts as a barrier to the neutralizing effect of saliva, thereby encouraging demineralization and destruction.

Saliva is the mouth's main defence against dental disease, buffering acid production and helping to wash away sugars. Furthermore, saliva supplies calcium and phosphate, which accelerate the process of remineralization. At night, reduced salivary flow increases the vulnerability of teeth to attack.

Many factors influence the initiation and progression of caries. Some teeth are simply less resistant to attack than others and this is unlikely to be due to poor maternal diet during pregnancy or after delivery, particularly in developed countries where severe malnutrition is rare. It is the interaction of local factors (saliva, plaque and the type, frequency and duration of dietary sugar intake) around the tooth that exerts the strongest influence on the severity of acid attack. Sugars are the most important dietary cause of caries, and a reduction in the amount and frequency of consumption of sugars is strongly recommended (2).

RELATIONSHIP BETWEEN DIET AND DENTAL CARIES

Diet and nutrition are relevant to dental health during the first year of life in two ways. First, before teeth appear, the deciduous dentition continues to develop within the jaws and calcification of the permanent dentition begins. Thus, good general nutrition is of some importance to both developing dentitions, and vitamin D supplementation of vitamin D-deficient pregnant women and children will reduce the occurrence of defective tooth structure (3). Second, the first teeth begin to appear at about 6 months of age, and the frequency and duration of exposure of these new teeth to sugars is highly significant in determining whether or not they develop carious lesions; this is more important than any pre-eruptive nutritional effects (4).

Added sugars are the primary culprits in the formation of dental caries. These are the sugars added during manufacturing, cooking or before consumption, found principally in confectionery, soft drinks, cakes, biscuits and table sugar, which are frequently eaten between meals as snacks and drinks. Sucrose is the most cariogenic sugar but glucose, fructose and maltose are only slightly less so. Sugars present in fresh fruits and vegetables and in starchy foods are not an important cause of tooth decay. Under normal dietary conditions, milk sugar (lactose) is not cariogenic. Breastfeeding is strongly encouraged by the dental profession, as breastfed babies tend to have a lower prevalence of dental caries than babies fed by bottle, probably because of the lack of opportunity to add sugar, and the lower use of reservoir feeders and comforters containing sugary drinks *(4)*. Human milk has been associated with the development of dental caries, but this is only when breastfeeding is prolonged (over 1 year) and preventive measures, such as brushing with fluoridated toothpaste, are not taken. Even then, development of dental caries is uncommon *(2)*. Incorrect feeding practices, in particular the addition of sweetened solids to milk, the bottle feeding of sweetened beverages, and the practice of sweetening pacifiers with honey or jam, are strongly associated with the development of nursing caries. It is therefore essential to establish good dietary practices, including the limited use of sugar, during the complementary feeding period (see Box 8).

Paediatric medicines with added sugars are implicated in dental caries. The trend to eliminate unnecessary sugars from all medicines should continue and, as far as possible, all paediatric medicines should be sugar-free.

PREVENTION OF DENTAL CARIES

Fluoride
Fluoride helps protect against decay by enhancing remineralization and by altering the structure of the tooth so that the surface is less soluble. It also reduces acid production, and thereby demineralization, by reducing bacterial metabolism. Fluoride can be supplied to the tooth either by ingestion, such as through drinking water (systemic application) or by direct application (topical application) to the tooth surface, such as in toothpaste.

Systemic application
Water fluoridation should be encouraged when drinking-water is fluoride-deficient (< 0.7 ml/litre) and there is a problem of dental caries. A large number of studies carried out worldwide have shown that water fluoridation at the optimal level leads to a significant reduction in caries *(5)*. The optimal level varies with climatic temperature, and is 1 part per million in

---

Box 8. The causes and prevention of dental caries

Characteristics of food and drink that contribute to the cariogenic process
- The frequency of intake of sucrose and /or other fermentable carbohydrates.
- The quantity of acid produced from a food/drink at the tooth surface.
- The amount of time that a food/drink remains in the mouth.
- The capacity to induce the formation of dental plaque.

Dietary advice
- To prevent dental caries during nursing, bottle feeding should be discouraged.
- Fruit juices and sweetened drinks, including tea, should not be given in a feeding bottle or reservoir feeder for the child to hold, especially at night.
- Sugary, fizzy drinks are not recommended.
- Pacifiers should be avoided.
- Advice should be aimed at reducing the amount and frequency of sugar consumption.
- Parents should be aware that the presentation of commercial foods as "free of added sugars" does not equate to "low in sugar". For example, sugars in concentrated fruit juices are equally as cariogenic as added sugars.
- Parents should be made aware of the sugar content of both sweet and savoury products.

---

temperate climates. Water fluoridation is the most effective means of preventing caries in children, provided a community has a piped water supply *(6)*. Systemic fluoridation can also be achieved through salt, milk and dietary supplementation.

In the absence of water fluoridation or the use of fluoridated salt or milk, fluoride dietary supplements may be given to children. Many trials have demonstrated their effectiveness, although the trend now is to target their use at high-risk groups and not to use dietary fluoride supplements as a public health measure *(5)*. Recommended dosages vary between countries, but in those where there is a high level of caries in the primary dentition, many dentists prefer a dosage regimen similar to that used in the United Kingdom since 1981 (Table 46).

Topical application
If possible, infants should visit the dentist at about 6 months of age, and definitely by 2 years of age, so that preventive advice can be given. Once

Table 46. Current dosage schedule for fluoride tablet supplements in the United Kingdom in relation to fluoride concentration in drinking-water

Fluoride in drinking-water (mg/litre)	Fluoride dosage (mg/day) by age group		
	6 months to 2 years	2–4 years	4–16 years
< 0.3	0.25	0.50	1.00
0.3–0.7	0.0	0.25	0.50
> 0.7	0.0	0.0	0.0

Source: World Health Organization *(5)*.

teeth have appeared they should be cleaned gently twice a day with a small toothbrush. The daily use of a fluoride toothpaste is an extremely effective method of delivering fluoride to the tooth surface and thereby preventing caries. Brushing also removes bacteria, thus helping to reduce the risk of periodontal disease.

No more than a smear or a *small* pea-sized amount of fluoride toothpaste is required. In many countries children's toothpastes are available, and can be recommended up to the age of 5 years. All children up to the age of at least 8 years will need assistance and supervision when cleaning their teeth.

Water fluoridation and fluoride toothpaste are very effective in preventing caries. For at-risk groups, other vehicles for applying fluoride such as fluoride drops, tablets, mouth rinses, gels and varnishes should be considered *(7)*.

The most cost-effective means of administering fluoride will depend on the resources available, the caries status of the community, and existing environmental sources of fluoride exposure. Health ministries are therefore advised to monitor the population's total fluoride exposure and the prevalence of both caries and fluorosis, in order to achieve the greatest benefits in terms of oral health *(5)*.

REFERENCES

1. MARTHALER, T.M. ORCA Symposium Report. The prevalence of dental caries in Europe 1990–1995. *Caries research*, **30**: 237–255 (1996).

2. RUGG-GUNN, A.J. British Society of Paediatric Dentistry: a policy document on sugars and the dental health of children. *International journal of paediatric dentistry*, **2**: 177–180 (1992).

3. COCKBURN, F. ET AL. Maternal vitamin D intake and mineral metabolism in mothers and their newborn infants. *British medical journal*, **2**: 11–14 (1980).

4. RUGG-GUNN, A.J. *Nutrition and dental health*. Oxford, Oxford University Press, 1993.

5. *Fluorides and oral health. Report of a WHO Expert Committee*. Geneva, World Health Organization, 1994 (WHO Technical Report Series, No. 846).

6. MURRAY, J.J. ET AL. *Fluorides in caries prevention*, 3rd ed. Oxford, Butterworth Heinemann, 1991.

7. *The scientific basis of dental health education: a policy document*, 4th ed. London, Health Education Authority, 1996.

Food safety

Safe food, clean water and good hygiene are essential to prevent diarrhoea and food- and water-borne diseases, which are a major cause of poor nutrition, stunting and recurrent illness.

Breastfeeding should be encouraged even where contamination of breast-milk is a concern, and mothers should be reassured that the risk from contamination is very small compared with the overall benefits of breastfeeding.

INTRODUCTION

Infants are exposed to food contaminants through breast-milk, infant formula and complementary foods, and are thus subject to the food safety problems experienced by the general population. Because infants and young children are especially susceptible, they are at greater risk of acquiring infections. When recurrent or persisting for a long period of time, infectious diseases have an adverse effect on nutritional status.

The scope of food safety problems is broad and diverse. It encompasses problems due to microorganisms (bacterial, parasitic and viral) and chemical hazards that may either be naturally present in foods or appear as contaminants as a result of pollution or poor agricultural practices. Physical hazards (such as glass and stones) have also proven to be an occasional problem.

MICROBIOLOGICAL CONTAMINATION

Nature of the problems

Contamination of food (including drinking-water) with microbial agents is one of the major causes of diarrhoeal diseases and ill health in infants and young children. Certain pathogens are opportunistic and affect mainly infants and young children. Some have particularly severe, others only mild, health consequences. Examples are *Aeromonas hydrophila* and other motile aeromonads, enterohaemorrhagic *Escherichia coli*, *Cryptosporidium parvum* and *Listeria monocytogenes*. A survey on enterohaemorrhagic *E. coli*, carried out in the United Kingdom from 1990 to 1998, showed that the incidence of this infection was highest in children under 5 years of age (8.8 cases per 100 000 inhabitants per year). Over 50% of those who developed haemolytic uraemic syndrome were less than 4 years old. The incidence of *Campylobacter* infections, highly prevalent in Europe, is also greatest among children under the age of 5 years. *Clostridium botulinum* is a specific problem in infants as the vegetative form of the pathogen can cause botulism, whereas in adults the bacterium itself is inoffensive and only the preformed toxin is dangerous. Infant botulism has often been associated with the consumption of honey. In addition to age other factors, such as the nutritional and health status of infants, determine the susceptibility of infants and young children to foodborne pathogens.

Health consequences

Foodborne diseases manifest themselves through a wide range of symptoms and signs, such as diarrhoea, vomiting, abdominal pain, fever and jaundice. They can cause severe and/or long-lasting damage to health, including acute, watery and bloody diarrhoeas (leading to severe dehydration and ulceration), meningitis, and chronic diseases affecting the renal, articular, cardiovascular, respiratory and immune systems. For example, children who are affected by enterohaemorrhagic *E. coli* can develop haemolytic uraemic syndrome, which sometimes leads to renal failure.

One of the serious implications of foodborne infections is their effect on nutritional status. Foodborne infections can lead to a reduction in food intake owing to anorexia. Poor food intake, aggravated by the loss of nutrients from vomiting, diarrhoea, malabsorption and fever over an extended period of time, will lead to nutritional deficiencies with serious consequences for growth and immune function in infants and children. Thus, an infant whose resistance is suppressed becomes vulnerable to other diseases and is subsequently caught in a vicious circle of malnutrition and infection.

Cause of foodborne diseases

In principle, all types of food may be implicated in foodborne diseases. The possibilities of cross-contamination, of contamination from raw materials or dirty surfaces/tools to cooked food or, to a lesser extent, contamination of food by food handlers, make almost any food a potential vehicle for any pathogen. However, certain foodborne diseases are more frequently associated with a specific food. Examples are given in Table 47.

The sources of food contamination are diverse. They include faeces, polluted water, flies, pests, domestic animals, unclean utensils and pots, food handlers, dust and dirt. Raw foods themselves are frequently a source of contaminants, as some may naturally harbour pathogens or derive them

Table 47. Examples of infectious diseases frequently associated with a specific food

Food	Examples of frequently associated foodborne diseases
Raw milk	Brucellosis, campylobacteriosis, enterohaemorrhagic *E. coli* infection, salmonellosis
Cheese made from raw milk	Listeriosis, *Staphylococcus aureus* intoxication, salmonellosis, brucellosis
Cream	Salmonellosis, *S. aureus* intoxication
Meat and meat products	Salmonellosis, campylobacteriosis, enterrohaemorrhagic *E. coli* infection, listeriosis, *S. aureus* intoxication, *Clostridium perfringens* gastroenteritis, botulism, taeniasis, trichinellosis
Poultry	Salmonellosis, campylobacteriosis
Egg and egg products	Salmonellosis
Fish and seafood	Salmonellosis, viral gastroenteritis, *Vibrio vulnificus* and *parahaemolyticus* infections, histamine intoxication
Rice, pasta and other cereal products	*Bacillus cereus* intoxication, *S. aureus* intoxication
Fruits and vegetables	Shigellosis, amoebiasis
Ice-cream	Salmonellosis, *S. aureus* intoxication
Pastry	Salmonellosis, *S. aureus* intoxication, *B. cereus* intoxication, *C. perfringens* gastroenteritis
Chocolate	Salmonellosis
Honey	Botulism
Drinking-water	Campylobacteriosis, crypstosporidiosis, giardiasis, amoebiasis, *E. coli* infection, shigellosis, typhoid fever, hepatitis A and E
Infant formula	*B. cereus* intoxication, salmonellosis

from infected animals. Moreover, during food preparation and storage, there is an added risk of cross-contamination as well as an opportunity for pathogenic bacteria to multiply. A careful analysis of foodborne diseases has shown that there are two particular errors in food preparation that increase this risk, as they permit the survival and growth of pathogens to disease-causing levels. These are:

- the preparation of food several hours before consumption, combined with its storage at temperatures favouring the growth of pathogens and/ or formation of toxins; and

- insufficient cooling or reheating of food to reduce or eliminate pathogens.

In addition to cases of food contamination in homes, about 2–12% of all outbreaks of foodborne diseases occur in day-care centres and kindergartens.

Prevalence of and trends in foodborne infections

The distribution of foodborne diseases varies according to region, lifestyle, food handling and food preparation practices, the health infrastructure and the degree of socioeconomic development. In the more industrialized parts of Europe, diseases such as campylobacteriosis, salmonellosis (except *S. typhi*), enterohaemorrhagic *E. coli* infection and listeriosis are more predominant, and there has been an increase in recent years. In the less industrialized parts of the Region, *Escherichia* spp., *Entamoeba histolytica*, hepatitis A and E and *Shigella* are cause for concern. Other pathogens, such as rotaviruses, *Crypstosporidium* and *Giardia lamblia,* are prevalent in all parts of Europe *(1,2)*.

Prevention and control of foodborne diseases

To prevent and control foodborne diseases in infants and young children, and to ensure the safety of complementary food, a clear understanding and observation of the rules of food hygiene is required, be it in the preparation of infant formula or solid foods. The general rules of hygiene are summarized in Box 9.

Sometimes, particularly when a problem with food safety is suspected, it may be necessary to conduct specific investigations into the food preparation practices of the caregivers and to identify specific errors in food preparation that may lead to food contamination. Investigations should include anthropological studies in order to identify any underlying sociocultural or economic factors that can lead to such errors.

Box 9. Basic principles for the preparation of safe food for infants and young children

Cook food thoroughly Many raw foods, notably poultry, raw milk and vegetables, are very often contaminated with disease-causing organisms. Thorough cooking will kill these organisms. For this purpose, all parts of the food must become steaming hot, which means they must reach a minimum temperature of 70 °C.

Avoid storing cooked food Prepare food for infants and young children freshly, and give it to them immediately after preparation when it is cool enough to eat. Foods prepared for infants and young children should preferably not be stored at all. If this is impossible, food could be stored only for the next meal, but kept cool (near or below 10 °C) or hot (near or above 60 °C). Stored food should be reheated thoroughly. Again, this means that all parts of the food must reach at least 70 °C.

Avoid contact between raw foodstuffs and cooked foods Cooked food can become contaminated through even the slightest contact with raw food. This cross-contamination can be direct but it can also be indirect and subtle, through hands, flies, utensils or unclean surfaces. Thus, hands should be washed after handling high-risk foods such as poultry. Similarly, utensils used for raw foods should be carefully washed before they are used again for cooked food. The addition of any new ingredients to cooked food may again introduce pathogenic organisms. In this case, food needs to be thoroughly cooked again.

Wash fruits and vegetables Fruits and vegetables, particularly if they are given to infants raw, must be washed carefully with safe water. If possible, vegetables and fruits should be peeled. Where such foods are likely to be heavily contaminated, for example when untreated waste water is used for irrigation or untreated nightsoil is used for soil fertilization, fruits and vegetables that cannot be peeled should be thoroughly cooked before they are given to infants.

Use safe water Safe water is just as important in preparing food for infants and young children as it is for drinking. Water used in preparing food should be boiled, unless the food to which the water is added has subsequently to be cooked, such as rice or potatoes. Remember that ice made with unsafe water will also be unsafe.

Wash hands repeatedly Wash hands thoroughly before you start preparing or serving food and after every interruption – especially if you have changed the baby, used the toilet or been in contact with animals. Domestic animals often harbour germs that can pass from hands to food.

Avoid feeding infants with a bottle Use a spoon and cup to give drinks and liquid foods to infants and young children. It is usually difficult to get bottles and teats completely clean. Spoons, cups, dishes and utensils used for preparing and feeding infants should be washed right after use. This will facilitate their thorough cleaning. If bottles and teats must be used, they should be thoroughly washed and boiled after every use.

Protect foods from insects, rodents and other animals Animals frequently carry pathogenic organisms and are potential sources of food contamination.

Store nonperishable foodstuffs in a safe place Keep pesticides, disinfecting agents or other toxic chemicals in labelled containers and separate from foodstuffs. To protect against rodents and insects, nonperishable foodstuffs should be stored in closed containers. Containers that have previously held toxic chemicals should not be used for storing foodstuffs.

Keep all food preparation premises meticulously clean Surfaces used for food preparation must be kept absolutely clean in order to avoid food contamination. Scraps of food and crumbs are potential reservoirs of germs and can attract insects and animals. Garbage should be kept safe in a covered place and be disposed of quickly.

Source: World Health Organization *(3)*.

Based on the information collected, caregivers should be trained in food safety. In this context, health care workers play an essential role and should be well trained and briefed to advise mothers and other caregivers in the safe handling of food (4).

CHEMICAL CONTAMINATION

Heavy metals

Foods and water contaminated with heavy metals pose risks to the health of infants and young children. In this section lead and cadmium will be highlighted. Table 48 summarizes food items that can be contaminated with these heavy metals.

Lead

Lead has an affinity for bone and can replace calcium. Gastrointestinal lead absorption and retention have been shown to vary widely, depending on the chemical conditions within the gastrointestinal lumen, a person's age and iron stores. Besides haemotoxicity and neural toxicity, anaemia and subnormal intelligence have been shown to result from long-term, low-level exposure to lead.

A significant number of household plumbing systems comprise lead pipes or solder. The majority of galvanized iron pipes contain lead and so lead may accumulate in the water. The lead intake of infants may therefore be influenced by the lead content of water, especially if it is given as a drink or added to infant formula or complementary foods. The lowest lead intakes are found in infants who are breastfed (5).

Cadmium

A number of European countries have reported intakes of cadmium in infants and children that are close to or exceed recommended limits.

Table 48. Potential food sources of lead and cadmium	
Lead	**Cadmium**
Milk, canned/fresh meat, kidney, liver, fish, molluscs, cereals, grains, canned/fresh fruit, fruit juice, spices, infant food, drinking-water, leaf vegetables, total diet	Kidney, molluscs, crustaceans, cereals, total diet

Source: World Health Organization (5).

Nevertheless, this is not thought to be serious as these limits are meant to be applied to regular intakes over a 50-year period *(6)*. The highest cadmium levels in drinking-water have been found in the Aral Sea region.

Dioxins and PCBs

Dioxin is the common name for 2,3,7,8-tetrachlorodibenzo-*p*-dioxin (TCDD) but is also used for the structurally and chemically related polychlorinated dibenzo-*p*-dioxins (PCDDs), polychlorinated dibenzofurans (PCDFs) and polychlorinated biphenyls (PCBs). TCDD can be taken up orally, is distributed freely in adipose tissue and is eliminated unchanged by excretion in faeces as well as by metabolism in the liver. Seven PCDDs and 10 PCDFs are considered toxic, and 11 PCBs have dioxin-like toxicity. The majority of toxic dioxins have been derived from industrial chlorination processes, incineration of municipal waste or the production of certain herbicides. All these compounds are fat-soluble and very stable and are therefore found in meat, milk, fish, human milk and human tissue *(5)*.

Breast-milk

According to the results of a European study in 1996 *(7)*, the levels of PCDDs and PCDFs in breast-milk have not increased since an earlier survey conducted in 1987 *(8)*. Indeed, in some countries the levels have fallen dramatically, by up to 50% compared to the 1987 study. The average infant intake of PCBs, PCDDs and PCDFs through breast-milk was estimated to be about 1–2 orders of magnitude below those causing adverse health effects. A greater risk of environmental PCB and dioxin exposure may occur during the prenatal period compared with exposure through breast-milk.

In some parts of central Asia levels of dioxins in breast-milk are high, especially in the Aral Sea region. TCDD concentrations of around 50 pg/g lipid in the milk of mothers from agricultural districts in Kazakhstan have been reported. These values are more than 10 times those found in milk from Swedish mothers *(9)*.

PCBs and dioxins are transported across the placenta and are also transferred into breast-milk, and there is evidence that these compounds can cause developmental neurotoxicity. Nevertheless, although relatively large amounts of PCBs and dioxins can be ingested by a breastfed infant, as yet no adverse effects have been found that outweigh the positive effects of breastfeeding on infant development.

Daily intakes of PCBs and dioxins (either on the basis of body weight or energy consumption) by breastfed infants are about 1–2 orders of magnitude higher than for the rest of the population. Compared with a lifetime exposure, however, only 5% of total PCB load is accumulated during a 6-month breastfeeding period. It is estimated that breastfeeding does not lead to significantly increased concentrations of PCBs in the adipose tissue of an infant, even though the most rapid gain in body fat occurs during infancy.

Mothers in highly contaminated areas, such as some parts of the central Asian republics, may be afraid to breastfeed through fear of feeding contaminated milk to their infants. Families may prefer to use infant formulas to reduce the risk of contamination, but this may expose infants to much greater risks from microbiologically unsafe water and the poor hygienic conditions that can result in diarrhoeal disease.

Foods

The lipophilic nature of dioxins results in their accumulation in the fat of meat and dairy products. Furthermore, surface contamination of plant foods and soil resulting from deposition of atmospheric emissions may be a significant direct source of dioxin.

The risk of exposure through breast-milk is much less than that during the fetal period. Therefore, risk management should be targeted towards pregnant women to limit their intake of contaminated foods *(10)*. For example, the Swedish Government advises pregnant and lactating women, and those who plan to become pregnant, not to eat fish from waters that are particularly polluted. It also recommends that nursing women should not lose large amounts of weight abruptly because this may mobilize contaminants that are potentially stored in fat *(11)*.

Strategies

Health experts and those concerned with the environment should continue to recommend breast-milk because of its benefits for the growth and development of the infant. Furthermore, certain practices such as trimming fat from meat, consuming low-fat dairy products, and simply cooking food can substantially reduce exposure to dioxin compounds. Nevertheless, primary preventive strategies to reduce the release of these chemicals into the environment provide the most effective way of minimizing exposure.

Nitrates, nitrites and methaemoglobinaemia

The toxicity of nitrate to humans is mainly attributable to its reduction to nitrite. Nitrite is especially harmful because it is involved in the oxidation of haemoglobin to methaemoglobin, which is unable to transport oxygen to the tissues. Because of their sensitivity to oxidizing agents, infants are particularly sensitive to poisons such as nitrites, and are thus more susceptible to the development of methaemoglobinaemia than older children and adults. Most clinical cases of methaemoglobinaemia therefore occur in infants under 3 months of age.

Drinking-water is the major source of nitrate for children, and methaemoglobinaemia often occurs when infants have consumed water with a high nitrate content. Intensification of farming is the principal cause of the increase in nitrate levels of groundwater. Water standards for nitrate (< 50 mg/litre) or nitrite (< 3 mg/litre) appear adequate for protection against methaemoglobinaemia *(12)*, but much higher levels may be present in the water in some areas of the former Soviet Union, including the central Asian republics *(13)*. Vegetables and fruits may also contain high nitrate concentrations and methaemoglobinaemia has been reported after consuming home-prepared spinach purée, carrot soup and juice.

Mycotoxins: aflatoxin

Aflatoxin has been reported in breast-milk, cow's milk, infant foods based on milk and especially in dairy products in south-east Kazakhstan. Although aflatoxin concentrations in infant formulas were found to be within acceptable limits for most countries, levels must be carefully evaluated because of the potentially negative effects of even very small amounts of aflatoxin on the growing infant *(6)*. Commercial formulas must be analysed regularly for the possible risk of aflatoxin contamination *(14)*, and human milk is safer than commercial formulas because of the lower risk of aflatoxin contamination.

Pesticides: DDT and hexachlorobenzene

Intrauterine exposure, in addition to breastfeeding, may account for the accumulation of fat-soluble pesticides in the adipose tissue of infants, notably DDT and hexachlorobenzene that may be present in food and breast-milk. DDT is still used in Kazakhstan, Tajikistan and Turkmenistan *(15)*. It is fat-soluble, and measurable concentrations are still reported by some countries in pork, beef and chicken fat as well as in milk and milk products *(6)*. The use of hexachlorobenzene as a fungicide on cereals has led to its appearance in milk and dairy products and in human milk owing to its fat solubility. A survey in Kazakhstan measured levels of hexachlorobenzene in breast-milk that were among the highest reported in the literature so far *(16)*.

Radioactive irradiation

During the Chernobyl accident, a great number of radionuclides were released into the atmosphere. The most important concerning the risk of ingestion by humans were iodine-131 (in the short term), cesium-134 and cesium-137 *(6)*. The Chernobyl breakdown resulted in an increase in childhood thyroid cancer and haematological disorders in Belarus and the Moscow region. The risk of radioactive iodine uptake is much higher in the presence of iodine deficiency, and therefore strong efforts to reduce the prevalence of iodine deficiency in mothers and children should be made to reduce the risk of thyroid cancers as seen after Chernobyl.

REFERENCES

1. TODD, E.C.D. Epidemiology of foodborne diseases: a worldwide review. *World health statistics quarterly*, **59**: 30–50 (1997).
2. MOTARJEMI, Y. & KÄFERSTEIN, F.K. Global estimation of foodborne diseases. *World health statistics quarterly*, **59**: 5–11 (1997).
3. *Health surveillance and management procedures for food-handling personnel: report of a WHO consultation.* Geneva, World Health Organization, 1989 (WHO Technical Report Series, No. 785).
4. ADAMS, M. & MOTARJEMI, Y. *Basic food safety for health workers.* Geneva, World Health Organization, 1999 (document WHO/SDE/PHE/FOS/99.1).
5. Lead, cadmium and mercury. *In*: *Trace elements in human nutrition and health*. Geneva, World Health Organization, 1996.
6. WHO EUROPEAN CENTRE FOR ENVIRONMENT AND HEALTH. *Concern for Europe's tomorrow: health and the environment in the WHO European Region*. Stuttgart, Wissenschaftliche Verlagsgesellschaft mbH, 1995, pp. 241–276.
7. WHO EUROPEAN CENTRE FOR ENVIRONMENT AND HEALTH. *Levels of PCBs, PCDDs and PCDFs in human milk. Second round of WHO-coordinated exposure study.* Copenhagen, WHO Regional Office for Europe, 1996 (document EUR/ICP/EHPM 02 03 05; Environmental Health in Europe, No. 3).
8. GRANDJEAN, P. ET AL., ED. *Assessment of health risks in infants associated with exposure to PCBs, PCDDs and PCDFs in breast milk. Report on a WHO Working Group.* Copenhagen, WHO Regional Office for Europe, 1988 (document EUR/ICP/CEH 533; Environmental Health Series, No. 29).
9. JENSEN, S. ET AL. Environment pollution and child health in the Aral Sea region in Kazakhstan. *Science of the total environment*, **206**: 187–193 (1997).

10. Schutz, D. et al. *GEMS/Food International Dietary Survey: infant exposure to certain organochlorine contaminants from breast milk – a risk assessment*. Geneva, World Health Organization, 1998 (document WHO/FSF/FOS/98.4).

11. Slorach, S. Measurements to reduce health risks from mercury and other chemical contaminants in fish. *Var föda*, **44**: 163–170 (1992).

12. *Guidelines for drinking-water quality*, 2nd ed. *Addendum to Vol. 2*. Geneva, World Health Organization, 1998 (document WHO/EOS/ 98.1), p. 63.

13. Fan, A.M. & Steinberg, V.E. Health implications of nitrate and nitrite in drinking water: an update on methemoglobinemia occurrence and reproductive and developmental toxicity. *Regulatory toxicology and pharmacology*, **23**: 35–43 (1996).

14. Aksit, S. et al. Aflatoxin: is it a neglected threat for formula-fed infants? *Acta paediatrica japonica*, **39**: 34–36 (1997).

15. Lederman, S.A. *Environmental contaminants and their significance for breastfeeding in the central Asian republics*. San Diego, CA, Wellstart International, 1993.

16. Hooper, K. et al. Analysis of breast milk to assess exposure to chlorinated contaminants in Kazakhstan: PCBs and organochlorine pesticides in southern Kazakhstan. *Environmental health perspectives*, **105**: 1254 (1997).

The International Code of Marketing of Breast-milk Substitutes and subsequent relevant resolutions of the World Health Assembly

INTERNATIONAL CODE OF MARKETING OF BREAST-MILK SUBSTITUTES

The Member States of the World Health Organization:

Affirming the right of every child and every pregnant and lactating woman to be adequately nourished as a means of attaining and maintaining health;

Recognizing that infant malnutrition is part of the wider problems of lack of education, poverty, and social injustice;

Recognizing that the health of infants and young children cannot be isolated from the health and nutrition of women, their socioeconomic status and their roles as mothers;

Conscious that breastfeeding is an unequalled way of providing ideal food for the healthy growth and development of infants; that it forms a unique biological and emotional basis for the health of both mother and child; that the anti-infective properties of breast-milk help to protect infants against disease; and that there is an important relationship between breastfeeding and child-spacing;

Recognizing that the encouragement and protection of breastfeeding is an important part of the health, nutrition and other social measures required to promote healthy growth and development of infants and young children; and that breastfeeding is an important aspect of primary health care;

Considering that when mothers do not breastfeed, or only do so partially, there is a legitimate market for infant formula and for suitable ingredients from which to prepare it; that all these products should accordingly be made accessible to those who need them through commercial or noncommercial distribution systems; and that they should not be marketed or distributed in ways that may interfere with the protection and promotion of breastfeeding;

Recognizing further that inappropriate feeding practices lead to infant malnutrition, morbidity and mortality in all countries, and that improper practices in the marketing of breast-milk substitutes and related products can contribute to these major public health problems;

Convinced that it is important for infants to receive appropriate complementary foods, usually when the infant reaches four to six months of age, and that every effort should be made to use locally available foods; and convinced, nevertheless, that such complementary foods should not be used as breast-milk substitutes;

Appreciating that there are a number of social and economic factors affecting breastfeeding, and that, accordingly, governments should develop social support systems to protect, facilitate and encourage it, and that they should create an environment that fosters breastfeeding, provides appropriate family and community support, and protects mothers from factors that inhibit breastfeeding;

Affirming that health care systems, and the health professionals and other health workers serving in them, have an essential role to play in guiding infant feeding practices, encouraging and facilitating breastfeeding, and providing objective and consistent advice to mothers and families about the superior value of breastfeeding, or, where needed, on the proper use of infant formula, whether manufactured industrially or home-prepared;

Affirming further that educational systems and other social services should be involved in the protection and promotion of breastfeeding, and in the appropriate use of complementary foods;

Aware that families, communities, women's organizations and other nongovernmental organizations have a special role to play in the protection and promotion of breastfeeding and in ensuring the support needed by pregnant women and mothers of infants and young children, whether breastfeeding or not;

Affirming the need for governments, organizations of the United Nations system, nongovernmental organizations, experts in various related disciplines, consumer groups and industry to cooperate in activities aimed at the improvement of maternal, infant and young child health and nutrition;

Recognizing that governments should undertake a variety of health, nutrition and other social measures to promote healthy growth and development of infants and young children, and that this Code concerns only one aspect of these measures;

Considering that manufacturers and distributors of breast-milk substitutes have an important and constructive role to play in relation to infant feeding, and in the promotion of the aim of this Code and its proper implementation;

Affirming that governments are called upon to take action appropriate to their social and legislative framework and their overall development objectives to give effect to the principles and aim of this Code, including the enactment of legislation, regulations or other suitable measures;

Believing that, in the light of the foregoing considerations, and in view of the vulnerability of infants in the early months of life and the risks involved in inappropriate feeding practices, including the unnecessary and improper use of breast-milk substitutes, the marketing of breast-milk substitutes requires special treatment, which makes usual marketing practices unsuitable for these products;

THEREFORE:

The Member States hereby agree the following articles which are recommended as a basis for action.

Article 1. Aim of the Code
The aim of this Code is to contribute to the provision of safe and adequate nutrition for infants, by the protection and promotion of breastfeeding, and by ensuring the proper use of breast-milk substitutes, when these are necessary, on the basis of adequate information and through appropriate marketing and distribution.

Article 2. Scope of the Code
The Code applies to the marketing, and practices related thereto, of the following products: breast-milk substitutes, including infant formula; other milk products, foods and beverages, including bottle-fed complementary foods, when marketed or otherwise represented to be suitable, with or without modification, for use as a partial or total replacement of breast-milk; and feeding bottles and teats. It also applies to their quality and availability, and to information concerning their use.

Article 3. Definitions
For the purposes of this Code:

"Breast-milk substitute" means any food being marketed or otherwise represented as a partial or total replacement for breast-milk, whether or not suitable for that purpose.

"Complementary food" means any food, whether manufactured or locally prepared, suitable as a complement to breast-milk or to infant formula, when either becomes insufficient to satisfy the nutritional requirements of the infant. Such food is also commonly called "weaning food" or "breast-milk supplement".

"Container" means any form of packaging of products for sale as a normal retail unit, including wrappers.

"Distributor" means a person, corporation or any other entity in the public or private sector engaged in the business (whether directly or indirectly) of marketing at the wholesale or retail level a product within the scope of this Code. A "primary distributor" is a manufacturer's sales agent, representative, national distributor or broker.

"Health care system" means governmental, nongovernmental or private institutions or organizations engaged, directly or indirectly, in health care for mothers, infants and pregnant women; and nurseries or childcare institutions. It also includes health workers in private practice. For the purposes of this Code, the health care system does not include pharmacies or other established sales outlets.

"Health worker" means a person working in a component of such a health care system, whether professional or nonprofessional, including voluntary, unpaid workers.

"Infant formula" means a breast-milk substitute formulated industrially in accordance with applicable Codex Alimentarius standards, to satisfy the normal nutritional requirements of infants up to between four and six months of age, and adapted to their physiological characteristics. Infant formula may also be prepared at home, in which case it is described as "home-prepared".

"Label" means any tag, brand, mark, pictorial or other descriptive matter, written, printed, stencilled, marked, embossed or impressed on, or attached to, a container (see above) of any products within the scope of this Code.

"Manufacturer" means a corporation or other entity in the public or private sector engaged in the business or function (whether directly or through an agent or through an entity controlled by or under contract with it) of manufacturing a product within the scope of this Code.

"Marketing" means product promotion, distribution, selling, advertising, product public relations, and information services.

"Marketing personnel" means any persons whose functions involve the marketing of a product or products coming within the scope of this Code.

"Samples" means single or small quantities of a product provided without cost.

"Supplies" means quantities of a product provided for use over an extended period, free or at a low price, for social purposes, including those provided to families in need.

Article 4. Information and education

4.1 Governments should have the responsibility to ensure that objective and consistent information is provided on infant and young child feeding for use by families and those involved in the field of infant and young child nutrition. This responsibility should cover either the planning, provision, design and dissemination of information, or their control.

4.2 Informational and educational materials, whether written, audio, or visual, dealing with the feeding of infants and intended to reach pregnant women and mothers of infants and young children, should include clear information on all the following points: (*a*) the benefits and superiority of breastfeeding; (*b*) maternal nutrition, and the preparation for and maintenance of breastfeeding; (*c*) the negative effect on breastfeeding of introducing partial bottle feeding; (*d*) the difficulty of reversing the decision not to breastfeed; and (*e*) where needed, the proper use of infant formula, whether manufactured industrially or home-prepared. When such materials contain information about the use of infant formula, they should include the social and financial implications of its use; the health hazards of inappropriate foods or feeding methods; and, in particular, the health hazards of unnecessary or improper use of infant formula and other breast-milk substitutes. Such materials should not use any pictures or text which may idealize the use of breast-milk substitutes.

4.3 Donations of informational or educational equipment or materials by manufacturers or distributors should be made only at the request and with the written approval of the appropriate government authority or within guidelines given by governments for this purpose. Such equipment or materials may bear the donating company's name or logo, but should not refer to a proprietary product that is within the scope of this Code, and should be distributed only through the health care system.

Article 5. The general public and mothers

5.1 There should be no advertising or other form of promotion to the general public of products within the scope of this Code.

5.2 Manufacturers and distributors should not provide, directly or indirectly, to pregnant women, mothers or members of their families, samples of products within the scope of this Code.

5.3 In conformity with paragraphs 1 and 2 of this Article, there should be no point-of-sale advertising, giving of samples, or any other promotion device to induce sales directly to the consumer at the retail level, such as special displays, discount coupons, premiums, special sales, loss leaders and tie-in sales, for products within the scope of this Code. This provision should not restrict the establishment of pricing policies and practices intended to provide products at lower prices on a long-term basis.

5.4 Manufacturers and distributors should not distribute to pregnant women or mothers of infants and young children any gifts of articles or utensils which may promote the use of breast-milk substitutes or bottle feeding.

5.5 Marketing personnel, in their business capacity, should not seek direct or indirect contact of any kind with pregnant women or with mothers of infants and young children.

Article 6. Health care systems

6.1 The health authorities in Member States should take appropriate measures to encourage and protect breastfeeding and promote the principles of this Code, and should give appropriate information and advice to health workers in regard to their responsibilities, including the information specified in Article 4.2.

6.2 No facility of a health care system should be used for the purpose of promoting infant formula or other products within the scope of this Code. This Code does not, however, preclude the dissemination of information to health professionals as provided in Article 7.2.

6.3 Facilities of health care systems should not be used for the display of products within the scope of this Code, for placards or posters concerning such products, or for the distribution of material provided by a manufacturer or distributor other than that specified in Article 4.3.

6.4 The use by the health care system of "professional service representatives", "mothercraft nurses" or similar personnel, provided or paid for by manufacturers or distributors, should not be permitted.

6.5 Feeding with infant formula, whether manufactured or home-prepared, should be demonstrated only by health workers, or other community workers if necessary; and only to the mothers or family members who need to use it; and the information given should include a clear explanation of the hazards of improper use.

6.6 Donations or low-price sales to institutions or organizations of supplies of infant formula or other products within the scope of this Code, whether for use in the institutions or for distribution outside them, may be made. Such supplies should only be used or distributed for infants who have to be fed on breast-milk substitutes. If these supplies are distributed for use outside the institutions, this should be done only by the institutions or organizations concerned. Such donations or low-price sales should not be used by manufacturers or distributors as a sales inducement.

6.7 Where donated supplies of infant formula or other products within the scope of this Code are distributed outside an institution, the institution or organization should take steps to ensure that supplies can be continued as long as the infants concerned need them. Donors, as well as institutions or organizations concerned, should bear in mind this responsibility.

6.8 Equipment and materials, in addition to those referred to in Article 4.3, donated to a health care system may bear a company's name or logo, but should not refer to any proprietary product within the scope of this Code.

Article 7. Health workers
7.1 Health workers should encourage and protect breastfeeding; and those who are concerned in particular with maternal and infant nutrition should make themselves familiar with their responsibilities under this Code, including the information specified in Article 4.2.

7.2 Information provided by manufacturers and distributors to health professionals regarding products within the scope of this Code should be restricted to scientific and factual matters, and such information should not imply or create a belief that bottle feeding is equivalent or superior to breastfeeding. It should also include the information specified in Article 4.2.

7.3 No financial or material inducements to promote products within the scope of this Code should be offered by manufacturers or distributors to health workers or members of their families, nor should these be accepted by health workers or members of their families.

7.4 Samples of infant formula or other products within the scope of this Code, or of equipment or utensils for their preparation or use, should not be provided to health workers except when necessary for the purpose of professional evaluation or research at the institutional level. Health workers should not give samples of infant formula to pregnant women, mothers of infants and young children, or members of their families.

7.5 Manufacturers and distributors of products within the scope of this Code should disclose to the institution to which a recipient health worker is affiliated any contribution made to him or on his behalf for fellowships, study tours, research grants, attendance at professional conferences, or the like. Similar disclosures should be made by the recipient.

Article 8. Persons employed by manufacturers and distributors

8.1 In systems of sales incentives for marketing personnel, the volume of sales of products within the scope of this Code should not be included in the calculation of bonuses, nor should quotas be set specifically for sales of these products. This should not be understood to prevent the payment of bonuses based on the overall sales by a company of other products marketed by it.

8.2 Personnel employed in marketing products within the scope of this Code should not, as part of their job responsibilities, perform educational functions in relation to pregnant women or mothers of infants and young children. This should not be understood as preventing such personnel from being used for other functions by the health care system at the request and with the written approval of the appropriate authority of the government concerned.

Article 9. Labelling

9.1 Labels should be designed to provide the necessary information about the appropriate use of the product, and so as not to discourage breastfeeding.

9.2 Manufacturers and distributors of infant formula should ensure that each container has a clear, conspicuous, and easily readable and understandable message printed on it, or on a label which cannot readily become separated from it, in an appropriate language, which includes all the following points: (*a*) the words "Important Notice" or their equivalent; (*b*) a statement of the superiority of breastfeeding; (*c*) a statement that the product should be used only on the advice of a health worker as to the need for its use and the proper method of use; (*d*) instructions for appropriate preparation, and a warning against the health hazards of inappropriate preparation. Neither the container nor the label should have pictures of infants, nor should they have other pictures or text which may idealize the use of infant formula. They may, however, have graphics for easy identification of the product as a breast-milk substitute and for illustrating methods of preparation. The terms "humanized", "maternalized" or similar terms should not be used. Inserts giving additional information about the product and its proper use, subject to the above conditions, may be included in the package or retail unit. When labels give instructions for modifying a product into infant formula, the above should apply.

9.3 Food products within the scope of this Code, marketed for infant feeding, which do not meet all the requirements of an infant formula, but which can be modified to do so, should carry on the label a warning that the unmodified product should not be the sole source of nourishment of an infant. Since sweetened condensed milk is not suitable for infant feeding, nor for use as a main ingredient of infant formula, its label should not contain purported instructions on how to modify it for that purpose.

9.4 The label of food products within the scope of this Code should also state all the following points: (*a*) the ingredients used; (*b*) the composition/ analysis of the product; (*c*) the storage conditions required; and (*d*) the batch number and the date before which the product is to be consumed, taking into account the climatic and storage conditions of the country concerned.

Article 10. Quality
10.1 The quality of products is an essential element for the protection of the health of infants and therefore should be of a high recognized standard.

10.2 Food products within the scope of this Code should, when sold or otherwise distributed, meet applicable standards recommended by the Codex Alimentarius Commission and also the Codex Code of Hygienic Practice for Foods for Infants and Children.

Article 11. Implementation and monitoring

11.1 Governments should take action to give effect to the principles and aim of this Code, as appropriate to their social and legislative framework, including the adoption of national legislation, regulations or other suitable measures. For this purpose, governments should seek, when necessary, the cooperation of WHO, UNICEF and other agencies of the United Nations system. National policies and measures, including laws and regulations, which are adopted to give effect to the principles and aim of this Code should be publicly stated, and should apply on the same basis to all those involved in the manufacture and marketing of products within the scope of this Code.

11.2 Monitoring the application of this Code lies with governments acting individually, and collectively through the World Health Organization as provided in paragraphs 6 and 7 of this Article. The manufacturers and distributors of products within the scope of this Code, and appropriate nongovernmental organizations, professional groups, and consumer organizations should collaborate with governments to this end.

11.3 Independently of any other measures taken for implementation of this Code, manufacturers and distributors of products within the scope of this Code should regard themselves as responsible for monitoring their marketing practices according to the principles and aim of this Code, and for taking steps to ensure that their conduct at every level conforms to them.

11.4 Nongovernmental organizations, professional groups, institutions, and individuals concerned should have the responsibility of drawing the attention of manufacturers or distributors to activities which are incompatible with the principles and aim of this Code, so that appropriate action can be taken. The appropriate governmental authority should also be informed.

11.5 Manufacturers and primary distributors of products within the scope of this Code should apprise each member of their marketing personnel of the Code and of their responsibilities under it.

11.6 In accordance with Article 62 of the Constitution of the World Health Organization, Member States shall communicate annually to the Director-General information on action taken to give effect to the principles and aim of this Code.

11.7 The Director-General shall report in even years to the World Health Assembly on the status of implementation of the Code; and shall, on request, provide technical support to Member States preparing national legislation or regulations, or taking other appropriate measures in implementation and furtherance of the principles and aim of this Code.

SUBSEQUENT RESOLUTIONS OF THE WORLD HEALTH ASSEMBLY

Resolution WHA33.32 (1980): Infant and young child feeding

The Thirty-third World Health Assembly,

Recalling resolutions WHA27.43 and WHA31.47 which in particular reaffirmed that breastfeeding is ideal for the harmonious physical and psychosocial development of the child, that urgent action is called for by governments and the Director-General in order to intensify activities for the promotion of breastfeeding and development of actions related to the preparation and use of weaning foods based on local products, and that there is an urgent need for countries to review sales promotion activities on baby foods and to introduce appropriate remedial measures, including advertisement codes and legislation, as well as to take appropriate supportive social measures for mothers working away from their homes during the lactation period;

Recalling further resolutions WHA31.55 and WHA32.42 which emphasized maternal and child health as an essential component of primary health care, vital to the attainment of health for all by the year 2000;

Recognizing that there is a close interrelationship between infant and young child feeding and social and economic development, and that urgent action by governments is required to promote the health and nutrition of infants, young children and mothers, *inter alia* through education, training and information in this field;

Noting that a joint WHO/UNICEF Meeting on Infant and Young Child Feeding was held from 9 to 12 October 1979, and was attended by representatives of governments, the United Nations system and technical agencies, nongovernmental organizations active in the area, the infant food industry and other scientists working in this field;

1. ENDORSES in their entirety the statement and recommendations made by the joint WHO/UNICEF Meeting, namely on the encouragement and

support of breastfeeding; the promotion and support of appropriate weaning practices; the strengthening of education, training and information; the promotion of the health and social status of women in relation to infant and young child feeding; and the appropriate marketing and distribution of breast-milk substitutes. This statement and these recommendations also make clear the responsibility in this field incumbent on the health services, health personnel, national authorities, women's and other nongovernmental organizations, the United Nations agencies and the infant-food industry, and stress the importance for countries to have a coherent food and nutrition policy and the need for pregnant and lactating women to be adequately nourished; the joint Meeting also recommended that "There should be an international code of marketing of infant formula and other products used as breast-milk substitutes. This should be supported by both exporting and importing countries and observed by all manufacturers. WHO and UNICEF are requested to organize the process for its preparation, with the involvement of all concerned parties, in order to reach a conclusion as soon as possible";

2. RECOGNIZES the important work already carried out by the World Health Organization and UNICEF with a view to implementing these recommendations and the preparatory work done on the formulation of a draft international code of marketing of breast-milk substitutes;

3. URGES countries which have not already done so to review and implement resolutions WHA27.43 and WHA32.42;

4. URGES women's organizations to organize extensive information dissemination campaigns in support of breastfeeding and healthy habits;

5. REQUESTS the Director-General:

(1) to cooperate with Member States on request in supervising or arranging for the supervision of the quality of infant foods during their production in the country concerned, as well as during their importation and marketing;

(2) to promote and support the exchange of information on laws, regulations, and other measures concerning marketing of breast-milk substitutes;

6. FURTHER REQUESTS the Director-General to intensify his activities for promoting the application of the recommendations of the joint WHO/UNICEF Meeting and, in particular:

(1) to continue efforts to promote breastfeeding as well as sound supplementary feeding and weaning practices as a prerequisite to healthy child growth and development;

(2) to intensify coordination with other international and bilateral agencies for the mobilization of the necessary resources for the promotion and support of activities related to the preparation of weaning foods based on local products in countries in need of such support and to collate and disseminate information on methods of supplementary feeding and weaning practices successfully used in different cultural settings;

(3) to intensify activities in the field of health education, training and information on infant and young child feeding, in particular through the preparation of training and other manuals for primary health care workers in different regions and countries;

(4) to prepare an international code of marketing of breast-milk substitutes in close consultation with Member States and with all other parties concerned including such scientific and other experts whose collaboration may be deemed appropriate, bearing in mind that:

(*a*) the marketing of breast-milk substitutes and weaning foods must be viewed within the framework of the problems of infant and young child feeding as a whole;

(*b*) the aim of the code should be to contribute to the provision of safe and adequate nutrition for infants and young children, and in particular to promote breastfeeding and ensure, on the basis of adequate information, the proper use of breast-milk substitutes, if necessary;

(*c*) the code should be based on existing knowledge of infant nutrition;

(*d*) the code should be governed *inter alia* by the following principles:

(i) the production, storage and distribution, as well as advertising, of infant feeding products should be subject to national legislation or regulations, or other measures as appropriate to the country concerned;

(ii) relevant information on infant feeding should be provided by the health care system of the country in which the product is consumed;

(iii) products should meet international standards of quality and presentation, in particular those developed by the Codex Alimentarius Commission, and their labels should clearly inform the public of the superiority of breastfeeding;

(5) to submit the code to the Executive Board for consideration at its sixty-seventh session and for forwarding with its recommendations to the Thirty-fourth World Health Assembly, together with proposals regarding its promotion and implementation, either as a regulation in the sense of Articles 21 or 22 of the Constitution of the World Health Organization or as a recommendation in the sense of Article 23, outlining the legal and other implications of each choice;

(6) to review the existing legislation in different countries for enabling and supporting breastfeeding, especially by working mothers, and to strengthen the Organization's capacity to cooperate on the request of Member States in developing such legislation;

(7) to submit to the Thirty-fourth World Health Assembly, in 1981, and thereafter in even years, a report on the steps taken by WHO to promote breastfeeding and to improve infant and young child feeding, together with an evaluation of the effect of all measures taken by WHO and its Member States.

Resolution WHA34.22 (1981): International Code of Marketing of Breast-milk Substitutes

The Thirty-fourth World Health Assembly,

Recognizing the importance of sound infant and young child nutrition for the future health and development of the child and adult;

Recalling that breastfeeding is the only natural method of infant feeding and that it must be actively protected and promoted in all countries;

Convinced that governments of Member States have important responsibilities and a prime role to play in the protection and promotion of breastfeeding as a means of improving infant and young child health;

Aware of the direct and indirect effects of marketing practices for breast-milk substitutes on infant feeding practices;

Convinced that the protection and promotion of infant feeding, including the regulation of the marketing of breast-milk substitutes, affect infant and young child health directly and profoundly, and are a problem of direct concern to WHO;

Having considered the draft prepared by the Director-General and forwarded to it by the Executive Board;

Expressing its gratitude to the Director-General and to the Executive Director of the United Nations Children's Fund for all the steps they have taken in ensuring close consultation with Member States and with all other parties concerned in the process of preparing the draft International Code;

Having considered the recommendation made thereon by the Executive Board at its sixty-seventh session;

Confirming resolution WHA33.32, including the endorsement in their entirety of the statement and recommendations made by the joint WHO/UNICEF Meeting on Infant and Young Child Feeding held from 9 to 12 October 1979;

Stressing that the adoption of and adherence to the code is a minimum requirement and only one of several important actions required in order to protect healthy practices in respect of infant and young child feeding;

1. ADOPTS, in the sense of Article 23 of the Constitution, the International Code of Marketing of Breast-milk Substitutes annexed to the present resolution;

2. URGES all Member States:

(1) to give full and unanimous support to the implementation of the recommendations made by the joint WHO/UNICEF Meeting on Infant and Young Child Feeding and of the provisions of the International Code in its entirety as an expression of the collective will of the membership of the World Health Organization;

(2) to translate the International Code into national legislation, regulations or other suitable measures;

(3) to involve all concerned social and economic sectors and all other concerned parties in the implementation of the International Code and in the observance of the provisions thereof;

(4) to monitor the compliance with the Code;

3. DECIDES that the follow-up to and review of the implementation of this resolution shall be undertaken by regional committees, the Executive Board and the Health Assembly in the spirit of resolution WHA33.17;

4. REQUESTS the FAO/WHO Codex Alimentarius Commission to give full consideration, within the framework of its operational mandate, to action it might take to improve the quality standards of infant foods, and to support and promote the implementation of the International Code;

5. REQUESTS the Director-General:

(1) to give all possible support to Member States, as and when requested, for the implementation of the International Code, and in particular in the preparation of national legislation and other measures related thereto in accordance with operative subparagraph 6(6) of resolution WHA33.32;

(2) to use his good offices for the continued cooperation with all parties concerned in the implementation and monitoring of the International Code at country, regional and global levels;

(3) to report to the Thirty-sixth World Health Assembly on the status of compliance with and implementation of the Code at country, regional and global levels;

(4) based on the conclusions of the status report, to make proposals, if necessary, for revision of the text of the Code and for the measures needed for its effective application.

Resolution WHA35.26 (1982): International Code of Marketing of Breast-milk Substitutes

The Thirty-fifth World Health Assembly,

Recalling resolution WHA33.32 on infant and young child feeding and resolution WHA34.22 adopting the International Code of Marketing of Breast-milk Substitutes;

Conscious that breastfeeding is the ideal method of infant feeding and should be promoted and protected in all countries;

Concerned that inappropriate infant feeding practices result in greater incidence of infant mortality, malnutrition and disease, especially in conditions of poverty and lack of hygiene;

Recognizing that commercial marketing of breast-milk substitutes for infants has contributed to an increase in artificial feeding;

Recalling that the Thirty-fourth World Health Assembly adopted an international code intended, *inter alia*, to deal with these marketing practices;

Noting that, while many Member States have taken some measures related to improving infant and young child feeding, few have adopted and adhered to the International Code as a "minimum requirement" and implemented it "in its entirety", as called for in resolution WHA34.22;

1. URGES Member States to give renewed attention to the need to adopt national legislation, regulations or other suitable measures to give effect to the International Code;

2. REQUESTS the Director-General:

(1) to design and coordinate a comprehensive programme of action to support Member States in their efforts to implement and monitor the Code and its effectiveness;

(2) to provide support and guidance to Member States as and when requested to ensure that the measures they adopt are consistent with the letter and spirit of the International Code;

(3) to undertake, in collaboration with Member States, prospective surveys, including statistical data of infant and young child feeding practices in the various countries, particularly with regard to the incidence and duration of breastfeeding.

Resolution WHA37.30 (1984): Infant and young child nutrition

The Thirty-seventh World Health Assembly,

Recalling resolutions WHA27.43, WHA31.47, WHA33.32, WHA34.22 and WHA35.26, which dealt with infant and young child feeding;

Recognizing that the implementation of the International Code of Marketing of Breast-milk Substitutes is one of the important actions required in order to promote healthy infant and young child feeding;

Recalling the discussion on infant and young child feeding at the Thirty-sixth World Health Assembly, which concluded that it was premature to revise the International Code at that time;

Having considered the Director-General's report, and noting with interest its contents;

Aware that many products unsuitable for infant feeding are being promoted for this purpose in many parts of the world, and that some infant foods are being promoted for use at too early an age, which can be detrimental to infant and young child health;

1. ENDORSES the Director-General's report;

2. URGES continued action by Member States, WHO, nongovernmental organizations and all other interested parties to put into effect measures to improve infant and young child feeding, with particular emphasis on the use of foods of local origin;

3. REQUESTS the Director-General:

(1) to continue and intensify collaboration with Member States in their efforts to implement and monitor the International Code of Marketing of Breast-milk Substitutes as an important measure at the national level;

(2) to support Member States in examining the problem of the promotion and use of foods unsuitable for infant and young child feeding, and ways of promoting the appropriate use of infant foods;

(3) to submit to the Thirty-ninth World Health Assembly a report on the progress in implementing this resolution, together with recommendations

for any other measures needed to further improve sound infant and young child feeding practices.

Resolution WHA39.28 (1986): Infant and young child feeding

The Thirty-ninth World Health Assembly,

Recalling resolutions WHA27.43, WHA31.47, WHA33.32, WHA34.22, WHA35.26 and WHA37.30 which dealt with infant and young child feeding;

Having considered the progress and evaluation report by the Director-General on infant and young child nutrition;

Recognizing that the implementation of the International Code of Marketing of Breast-milk Substitutes is an important contribution to healthy infant and young child feeding in all countries;

Aware that today, five years after the adoption of the International Code, many Member States have made substantial efforts to implement it, but that many products unsuitable for infant feeding are nonetheless being promoted and used for this purpose; and that sustained and concerted efforts will therefore continue to be necessary to achieve full implementation of and compliance with the International Code as well as the cessation of the marketing of unsuitable products and the improper promotion of breast-milk substitutes;

Noting with great satisfaction the guidelines concerning the main health and socioeconomic circumstances in which infants have to be fed on breast-milk substitutes, in the context of Article 6, paragraph 6, of the International Code;

Noting further the statement in the guidelines, paragraph 47: "Since the large majority of infants born in maternity wards and hospitals are full term, they require no nourishment other than colostrum during their first 24–48 hours of life – the amount of time often spent by a mother and her infant in such an institutional setting. Only small quantities of breast-milk substitutes are ordinarily required to meet the needs of a minority of infants in these facilities, and they should only be available in ways that do not interfere with the protection and promotion of breastfeeding for the majority";

1. ENDORSES the report of the Director-General;

2. URGES Member States:

(1) to implement the Code if they have not yet done so;

(2) to ensure that the practices and procedures of their health care systems are consistent with the principles and aim of the International Code;

(3) to make the fullest use of all concerned parties – health professional bodies, nongovernmental organizations, consumer organizations, manufacturers and distributors – generally, in protecting and promoting breastfeeding and, specifically, in implementing the Code and monitoring its implementation and compliance with its provisions;

(4) to seek the cooperation of manufacturers and distributors of products within the scope of Article 2 of the Code, in providing all information considered necessary for monitoring the implementation of the Code;

(5) to provide the Director-General with complete and detailed information on the implementation of the Code;

(6) to ensure that the small amounts of breast-milk substitutes needed for the minority of infants who require them in maternity wards are made available through the normal procurement channels and not through free or subsidized supplies;

3. REQUESTS the Director-General:

(1) to propose a simplified and standardized form for use by Member States to facilitate the monitoring and evaluation by them of their implementation of the Code and reporting thereon to WHO, as well as the preparation by WHO of a consolidated report covering each of the articles of the Code;

(2) to specifically direct the attention of Member States and other interested parties to the following:

(a) any food or drink given before complementary feeding is nutritionally required may interfere with the initiation or maintenance of breastfeeding and therefore should neither be promoted nor encouraged for use by infants during this period;

(b) the practice being introduced in some countries of providing infants with specially formulated milks (so-called "follow-up milks") is not necessary.

Resolution WHA41.11 (1988): Infant and young child nutrition

The Forty-first World Health Assembly,

Having considered the report by the Director-General on infant and young child nutrition;

Recalling resolutions WHA33.32, WHA34.22, and WHA39.28 on infant and young child feeding and nutrition, and resolutions WHA37.18 and WHA39.31 on the prevention and control of vitamin A deficiency and xerophthalmia, and of iodine deficiency disorders;

Concerned at continuing decreasing breastfeeding trends in many countries, and committed to the identification and elimination of obstacles to breastfeeding;

Aware that appropriate infant and young child nutrition could benefit from further broad national, community and family interventions;

1. COMMENDS governments, women's organizations, professional associations, consumer and other nongovernmental groups, and the food industry for their efforts to promote appropriate infant and young child nutrition, and encourages them, in cooperation with WHO, to support national efforts for coordinated nutrition programmes and practical action at country level to improve the health and nutrition of women and children;

2. URGES Member States:

(1) to develop or enhance national nutrition programmes, including multisectoral approaches, with the objective of improving the health and nutritional status of their populations, especially that of infants and young children;

(2) to ensure practices and procedures that are consistent with the aim and principles of the International Code of Marketing of Breast-milk Substitutes, if they have not already done so;

3. REQUESTS the Director-General to continue to collaborate with Member States, through WHO regional offices and in collaboration with other agencies of the United Nations system, especially FAO and UNICEF:

(1) in identifying and assessing the main nutrient and dietary problems, developing national strategies to deal with them, applying these strategies, and monitoring and evaluating their effectiveness;

(2) in establishing effective nutritional status surveillance systems in order to ensure that all the main variables which collectively determine nutritional status are properly addressed;

(3) in compiling, analysing, managing and applying information that they have gathered on the nutritional status of their populations;

(4) in monitoring, together with other maternal and child health indicators, changes in the prevalence and duration of full and supplemented breastfeeding with a view to improving breastfeeding rates;

(5) in developing recommendations regarding diet, including timely complementary feeding and appropriate weaning practices, which are appropriate to national circumstances;

(6) in providing legal and technical assistance, upon request from Member States, in the drafting and/or the implementation of national codes of marketing of breast-milk substitutes, or other similar instruments;

(7) in designing and implementing collaborative studies to assess the impact of measures taken to promote breastfeeding and child nutrition in Member States.

Resolution 43.3 (1990): Protecting, promoting and supporting breastfeeding

The Forty-third World Health Assembly,

Recalling resolutions WHA33.32, WHA34.22, WHA35.26, WHA37.30, WHA39.28 and WHA41.11 on infant and young child feeding and nutrition;

Having considered the report by the Director-General on infant and young child nutrition;

Reaffirming the unique biological properties of breast-milk in protecting against infections, in stimulating the development of the infant's own immune system, and in limiting the development of some allergies;

Recalling the positive impact of breastfeeding on the physical and emotional health of the mother, including its important contribution to child-spacing;

Convinced of the importance of protecting breastfeeding among groups and populations where it remains the infant-feeding norm, and promoting it where it is not, through appropriate information and support, as well as recognizing the special needs of working women;

Recognizing the key role in protecting and promoting breastfeeding played by health workers, particularly nurses, midwives and those in child health/family planning programmes, and the significance of the counselling and support provided by mothers' groups;

Recognizing that, in spite of resolution WHA39.28, free or low-cost supplies of infant formula continue to be available to hospitals and maternities, with adverse consequences for breastfeeding;

Reiterating its concern over the decreasing prevalence and duration of breastfeeding in many countries;

1. THANKS the Director-General for his report;

2. URGES Member States:

(1) to protect and promote breastfeeding, as an essential component of their overall food and nutrition policies and programmes on behalf of women and children, so as to enable all infants to be exclusively breastfed during the first four to six months of life;

(2) to promote breastfeeding, with due attention to the nutritional and emotional needs of mothers;

(3) to continue monitoring breastfeeding patterns, including traditional attitudes and practices in this regard;

(4) to enforce existing, or adopt new, maternity protection legislation or other suitable measures that will promote and facilitate breastfeeding among working women;

(5) to draw the attention of all who are concerned with planning and providing maternity services to the universal principles affirmed in the joint WHO/UNICEF statement on breast-feeding and maternity services that was issued in 1989;

(6) to ensure that the principles and aim of the International Code of Marketing of Breast-milk Substitutes and the recommendations contained in resolution WHA39.28 are given full expression in national health and nutritional policy and action, in cooperation with professional associations, women's organizations, consumer and other nongovermental groups, and the food industry;

(7) to ensure that families make the most appropriate choice with regard to infant feeding, and that the health system provides the necessary support;

3. REQUESTS the Director-General, in collaboration with UNICEF and other international and bilateral agencies concerned:

(1) to urge Member States to take effective measures to implement the recommendations included in resolution WHA39.28;

(2) to continue to review regional and global trends in breastfeeding patterns, including the relationship between breastfeeding and child-spacing;

(3) to support Member States, on request, in adopting measures to improve infant and young child nutrition, *inter alia* by collecting and disseminating information on relevant national action of interest to all Member States; and to mobilize technical and financial resources to this end.

Resolution WHA45.34 (1992): Infant and young child nutrition and status of implementation of the International Code of Marketing of Breast-milk Substitutes

The Forty-fifth World Health Assembly,

Having considered the report by the Director-General on infant and young child nutrition;

Recalling resolutions WHA33.32, WHA34.22, WHA35.26, WHA37.30 WHA39.28, WHA41.11 and WHA43.3 on infant and young child feeding and nutrition, appropriate feeding practices and related questions;

Reaffirming that the International Code of Marketing of Breast-milk Substitutes is a minimum requirement and only one of several important actions required in order to protect healthy practices in respect of infant and young child feeding;

Recalling that products that may be promoted as a partial or total replacement for breast-milk, especially when these are presented as suitable for bottle feeding, are subject to the provisions of the International Code;

Reaffirming that during the first four to six months of life no food or liquid other than breast-milk, not even water, is required to meet the normal infant's nutritional requirements, and that from the age of about six months infants should begin to receive a variety of locally available and safely prepared foods rich in energy, in addition to breast-milk, to meet their changing nutritional requirements;

Welcoming the leadership of the Executive Heads of WHO and UNICEF in organizing the "baby-friendly" hospital initiative, with its simultaneous focus on the role of health services in protecting, promoting and supporting breastfeeding and on the use of breastfeeding as a means of strengthening the contribution of health services to safe motherhood, child survival, and primary health care in general, and endorsing this initiative as a most promising means of increasing the prevalence and duration of breastfeeding;

Expressing once again its concern about the need to protect and support women in the workplace, for their own sakes but also in the light of their multiple roles as mothers and care-providers, *inter alia*, by applying existing legislation fully for maternity protection, expanding it to cover any women at present excluded or, where appropriate, adopting new measures to protect breastfeeding;

Encouraged by the steps being taken by infant-food manufacturers towards ending the donation or low-price sale of supplies of infant formula to maternity wards and hospitals, which would constitute a step towards full implementation of the International Code;

Being convinced that charitable and other donor agencies should exert great care in initiating, or responding to, requests for free supplies of infant foods;

Noting that the advertising and promotion of infant formula and the presentation of other products as breast-milk substitutes, as well as feeding-bottles and teats, may compete unfairly with breastfeeding which is the safest and lowest-cost method of nourishing an infant, and may exacerbate such competition and favour uninformed decision-making by interfering with the advice and guidance to be provided by the mother's physician or health worker;

Welcoming the generous financial and other contributions from a number of Member States that enabled WHO to provide technical support to countries wishing to review and evaluate their own experiences in giving effect to the International Code;

1. THANKS the Director-General for his report;

2. URGES Member States:

(1) to give full expression at national level to the operational targets contained in the Innocenti Declaration, namely:

(*a*) by appointing a national breastfeeding coordinator and establishing a multisectoral breastfeeding committee;

(*b*) by ensuring that every facility providing maternity services applies the principles laid down in the joint WHO/UNICEF statement on the role of maternity services in protecting, promoting and supporting breastfeeding;

(*c*) by taking action to give effect to the principles and aim of the International Code of Marketing of Breast-milk Substitutes and subsequent relevant Health Assembly resolutions in their entirety;

(*d*) by enacting legislation and adopting means for its enforcement to protect the breastfeeding rights of working women;

(2) to encourage and support all public and private health facilities providing maternity services so that they become "baby-friendly":

(*a*) by providing the necessary training in the application of the principles laid down in the joint WHO/UNICEF statement;

(*b*) by encouraging the collaboration of professional associations, women's organizations, consumer and other nongovernmental groups, the food industry, and other competent sectors in this endeavour;

(3) to take measures appropriate to national circumstances aimed at ending the donation or low-priced sale of supplies of breast-milk substitutes to health-care facilities providing maternity services;

(4) to use the common breastfeeding indicators developed by WHO, with the collaboration of UNICEF and other interested organizations and agencies, in evaluating the progress of their breastfeeding programmes;

(5) to draw upon the experiences of other Member States in giving effect to the International Code;

3. REQUESTS the Director-General:

(1) to continue WHO's productive collaboration with its traditional international partners, in particular UNICEF, as well as other concerned parties including professional associations, women's organizations, consumer groups and other nongovernmental organizations and the food industry, with a view to attaining the Organization's goals and objectives in infant and young child nutrition;

(2) to strengthen the Organization's network of collaborating centres, institutions and organizations in support of appropriate national action;

(3) to support Member States, on request, in elaborating and adapting guidelines on infant nutrition, including complementary feeding practices that are timely, nutritionally appropriate and biologically safe and in devising suitable measures to give effect to the International Code;

(4) to draw the attention of Member States and other intergovernmental organizations to new developments that have an important bearing on infant and young child feeding and nutrition;

(5) to consider, in collaboration with the International Labour Organization, the options available to the health sector and other interested sectors for reinforcing the protection of women in the workplace in view of their maternal responsibilities, and to report to a future Health Assembly in this regard;

(6) to mobilize additional technical and financial resources for intensi-
fied support to Member States.

Resolution WHA47.5 (1994): Infant and young child nutrition

The Forty-seventh World Health Assembly,

Having considered the report by the Director-General on infant and young
child nutrition;

Recalling resolutions WHA33.32, WHA34.22 WHA35.26, WHA37.30,
WHA39.28, WHA41.11, WHA43.3, WHA45.34, WHA46.7 concerning infant and young child nutrition, appropriate feeding practices and
related questions;

Reaffirming its support for all these resolutions and reiterating the recommendations to Member States contained therein;

Bearing in mind the superiority of breast-milk as the biological norm for
nourishing infants, and that a deviation from this norm is associated with
increased risks to the health of infants and mothers;

1. THANKS the Director-General for his report;

2. URGES Member States to take the following measures:

(1) to promote sound infant and young child nutrition, in keeping with
their commitment to the World Declaration for Nutrition, through
coherent effective intersectoral action, including:

(*a*) increasing awareness among health personnel, nongovernmental organizations, communities and the general public of the importance of
breastfeeding and its superiority to any other infant feeding method;

(*b*) supporting mothers in their choice to breastfeed by removing
obstacles and preventing interference that they may face in health
services, the workplace, or the community;

(*c*) ensuring that all health personnel concerned are trained in
appropriate infant and young child feeding practices, including

the application of the principles laid down in the joint WHO/ UNICEF statement on breastfeeding and the role of maternity services;

(*d*) fostering appropriate complementary feeding practices from the age of about six months, emphasizing continued breastfeeding and frequent feeding with safe and adequate amounts of local foods;

(2) to ensure that there are no donations of free or subsidized supplies of breast-milk substitutes and other products covered by the International Code of Marketing of Breast-milk Substitutes in any part of the health care system;

(3) to exercise extreme caution when planning, implementing or supporting emergency relief operations, by protecting, promoting and supporting breastfeeding for infants, and ensuring that donated supplies of breast-milk substitutes or other products covered by the scope of the International Code be given only if all the following conditions apply:

(*a*) infants have to be fed on breast-milk substitutes, as outlined in the guidelines concerning the main health and socioeconomic circumstances in which infants have to be fed on breast-milk substitutes;

(*b*) the supply is continued for as long as the infants concerned need it;

(*c*) the supply is not used as a sales inducement;

(4) to inform the labour sector, and employers' and workers' organizations, about the multiple benefits of breastfeeding for infants and mothers, and the implications for maternity protection in the workplace;

3. REQUESTS the Director-General:

(1) to use his good offices for cooperation with all parties concerned in giving effect to this and related resolutions of the Health Assembly in their entirety;

(2) to complete development of a comprehensive global approach and programme of action to strengthen national capacities for improving infant and young child feeding practices; including the development of

methods and criteria for national assessment of breastfeeding trends and practices;

(3) to support Member States, at their request, in monitoring infant and young child feeding practices and trends in health facilities and households, in keeping with new standard breastfeeding indicators;

(4) to urge Member States to initiate the Baby-friendly Hospital Initiative and to support them, at their request, in implementing this Initiative, particularly in their efforts to improve educational curricula and in-service training for all health and administrative personnel concerned;

(5) to increase and strengthen support to Member States, at their request, in giving effect to the principles and aim of the International Code and all relevant resolutions, and to advise Member States on a framework which they may use in monitoring their application, as appropriate to national circumstances;

(6) to develop, in consultation with other concerned parties and as part of WHO's normative function, guiding principles for the use in emergency situations of breast-milk substitutes or other products covered by the International Code which the competent authorities in Member States may use, in the light of national circumstances, to ensure the optimal infant-feeding conditions;

(7) to complete, in cooperation with selected research institutions, collection of revised reference data and the preparation of guidelines for their use and interpretation, for assessing the growth of breastfed infants;

(8) to seek additional technical and financial resources for intensifying WHO's support to Member States in infant feeding and in the implementation of the International Code and subsequent relevant resolutions.

Resolution WHA49.15 (1996): Infant and young child nutrition

The Forty-ninth World Health Assembly,

Having considered the summary of the report by the Director-General on infant feeding and young child nutrition;

Recalling resolutions WHA33.32, WHA34.22, WHA39.28 and WHA45.34 among others concerning infant and young child nutrition, appropriate feeding practices and other related questions;

Recalling and reaffirming the provisions of resolution WHA47.5 concerning infant and young child nutrition, including the emphasis on fostering appropriate complementary feeding practices;

Concerned that health institutions and ministries may be subject to subtle pressure to accept, inappropriately, financial or other support for professional training in infant and child health;

Noting the increasing interest in monitoring the application of the International Code of Marketing of Breast-milk Substitutes and subsequent relevant Health Assembly resolutions;

1. THANKS the Director-General for his report;

2. STRESSES the continued need to implement the International Code of Marketing of Breast-milk Substitutes, subsequent relevant resolutions of the Health Assembly, the Innocenti Declaration, and the World Declaration and Plan of Action for Nutrition;

3. URGES Member States to take the following measures:

(1) to ensure that complementary foods are not marketed for or used in ways that undermine exclusive and sustained breastfeeding;

(2) to ensure that the financial support for professionals working in infant and young child health does not create conflicts of interest, especially with regard to the WHO/UNICEF Baby-friendly Hospital Initiative;

(3) to ensure that monitoring the application of the International Code and subsequent relevant resolutions is carried out in a transparent, independent manner, free from commercial influence;

(4) to ensure that the appropriate measures are taken including health information and education in the context of primary health care, to encourage breastfeeding;

(5) to ensure that the practices and procedures of their health care systems are consistent with the principles and aims of the International Code of Marketing of Breast-milk Substitutes;

(6) to provide the Director-General with complete and detailed information on the implementation of the Code;

4. REQUESTS the Director-General to disseminate, as soon as possible, to Member States document WHO/NUT/96.4 (currently in preparation) on the guiding principles for feeding infants and young children during emergencies.

Prevention of mother-to-child transmission of HIV

WHO/UNICEF/UNAIDS STATEMENT ON CURRENT STATUS OF WHO/UNICEF/UNAIDS POLICY GUIDELINES, 3 SEPTEMBER 1999

A recent early report of evidence that HIV is less likely to be transmitted through exclusive breastfeeding does not warrant a change in existing WHO/UNICEF/UNAIDS policy.

In the last ten years, evidence has accumulated that HIV can be transmitted through breast-milk. WHO and UNAIDS currently estimate that a child breastfeeding from a mother who is HIV positive has a 15% risk of infection by this route. Every year 200 000 infants may acquire HIV in this way. Where resources permit, many HIV-positive mothers now choose to feed their babies artificially and to avoid breastfeeding altogether. In resource-poor settings, where the risk of artificial feeding may be particularly high, the decision for both individual mothers and policy-makers is more difficult. The situation has led in some settings to a loss of support for initiatives to promote breastfeeding and to some women avoiding breastfeeding even if they do know their HIV status.

In 1997, UNAIDS, WHO and UNICEF issued a joint policy statement on HIV and infant feeding, which stated that:

- as a general principle, in all populations, irrespective of HIV infection rates, breastfeeding should continue to be protected, promoted and supported;
- counselling for women who are aware of their HIV status should include the best available information on the benefits of breastfeeding, on the risk of HIV transmission through breastfeeding and on the risks and possible advantages associated with other methods of infant feeding; and
- it is, therefore, important that women be empowered to make fully informed decisions about infant feeding and that they be suitably supported in carrying them out.

In 1998, WHO, UNICEF and UNAIDS held a technical consultation on HIV and infant feeding and issued guidelines with a human rights perspective, based on the joint policy statement *(1,2)*. These guidelines call for a strengthening of initiatives to protect, promote and support breastfeeding among mothers who are HIV-negative or of unknown HIV status, and they include several infant-feeding options for consideration by HIV-positive mothers. These include:

- replacement feeding with commercial formula or home-prepared formula;
- breastfeeding in the way generally recommended;
- breastfeeding exclusively and stopping early;
- use of heat-treated expressed breast-milk; and
- wet-nursing.

In all cases there should be timely and adequate complementary feeding. There is no attempt to favour any one of these options over the others, as the principal recommendation is for mothers to receive counselling that will enable them to make a fully informed decision appropriate to their situation and resources. The responsibility of the policy-maker and health care manager is to provide the necessary support to enable mothers to make and carry out their choice, whether to breastfeed or to use replacement feeds.

The studies on which existing estimates of transmission are based do not distinguish between infants who are exclusively breastfed and those, usually the majority, who are both breastfed and receive other foods or drinks. A recently published early report *(3)* suggests that exclusive breastfeeding – that is, when an infant is given no other food or drink of any sort – may be less likely to transmit infection than mixed feeding, possibly because other foods can damage the infant's gut and make it easier for the virus to cross the intestinal mucosa. This report has raised the hopes of many health workers who are concerned about the adverse effects on child health of decreasing rates of breastfeeding. The question has been raised as to whether or not WHO/UNICEF/UNAIDS should revise its HIV and infant feeding recommendation.

The information contained in this early report is interesting and important. Because of limitations of the study size and design, however, firm conclusions cannot be drawn without further research. That such research should be conducted as a matter or urgency is clear and has been identified by WHO as a priority.

The current guidelines clearly indicate that for HIV-positive mothers who choose to breastfeed, the safest option is to breastfeed exclusively to minimize the risk of other childhood infections such as diarrhoea, using a good technique to reduce the risk of mastitis and nipple damage that could increase transmission of HIV. Stopping breastfeeding when the infant is 3–6 months old is an option to avoid late postnatal transmission, and at this older age the health hazards for the child, and the social difficulties for the mother associated with not breastfeeding, are fewer.

Short-term exclusive breastfeeding is already included in the WHO/UNICEF/UNAIDS guidelines as one of the feeding options. The information in the early report, if confirmed, would strengthen the case for choosing it as both feasible and effective. Nevertheless, there can be no justification for dropping replacement feeding as one of the options, for mothers who wish to use it, while there is any possibility of transmission of HIV through breast-milk.

The existing WHO/UNICEF/UNAIDS policy and guidelines remain appropriate according to existing scientific evidence, and there is no present indication that they should be changed. The guidelines accommodate all reasonable infant feeding options for mothers with HIV and support a fully informed choice, which will allow mothers to be provided with better information as it becomes available.

1. *HIV and infant feeding. Guidelines for decision-makers.* Geneva, World Health Organization, 1998 (document WHO/FRH/NUT 98.1).
2. *HIV and infant feeding. A guide for health care managers and supervisors.* Geneva, World Health Organization, 1998 (document WHO/FRH/NUT 98.2).
3. COUTSOUDIS, A. ET AL. Influence of infant-feeding patterns on early mother-to-child transmission of HIV-1 in Durban, South Africa: a prospective cohort study. *Lancet*, **354**: 471–476 (1999).

Infant feeding in Integrated Management of Childhood Illness

Integrated Management of Childhood Illness (IMCI) is an approach developed by WHO and UNICEF that provides basic care for the most common childhood illnesses, as well as preventive measures, and improved family and community practices related to child health. Its aims are to reduce deaths, reduce the frequency and severity of illness and disability among children, and contribute to improved growth and development.

The strategy combines aspects of treatment of prevalent diseases, nutrition, immunization and several other important influences on child health, including maternal health. Nutrition has been included as an important component because malnutrition is associated with over 50% of childhood deaths. In many settings, inadequate feeding practices have been identified as a major contributor to malnutrition. Given that most malnourished children are not treated in hospital, priority must be given to developing approaches to the prevention and management of malnutrition at home.

THE PROGRESS OF IMCI IN THE EUROPEAN REGION

The WHO Regional Office for Europe, in collaboration with other WHO programmes, UNICEF and numerous other agencies and institutions, is introducing the IMCI strategy into the European Region, and started in Kazakhstan in 1996. An initial pilot survey conducted for IMCI on the adaptation of infant and young child feeding recommendations found that lack of calories was not a significant problem. Maternal knowledge, however, represented a significant barrier to improvements in infant and young child feeding practices. Meals lacked variety and were of low frequency, the types of foods offered were not ideal, and the preparation of food and how it was given to the child could be improved. Nevertheless, mothers were very willing to try new suggestions. For example, advice on the inclusion of night breastfeeds was particularly well accepted, and even with minimal resources it was possible for mothers to find ways to improve the feeding of their children.

THE "FOOD BOX" ADAPTATION

A major part of the IMCI materials is on child feeding. This includes:
(*a*) *Assess the child's feeding*, with questions for assessing child feeding practices;

(*b*) *Food box*, with feeding recommendations for the sick and well child divided by age group; and (*c*) *Counsel the mother about feeding problems*, with recommendations for counselling mothers on specific feeding problems. These materials are referred to by health workers when assessing and counselling mothers on child feeding. The materials also include the *Counsel the mother* module used in training, which explains how to counsel the mother on feeding practices.

The following text and Box 1 give examples from Azerbaijan.

SOME OF THE COMMON PROBLEMS FOUND IN AZERBAIJAN
Up to 4 months

Ideal feeding pattern
exclusive breastfeeding.

Problem 1. Mother is not breastfeeding exclusively.
- She perceives she has not enough milk.
- She has been advised to use other foods/fluids.

Recommendations
- Give only breast-milk. Stop other foods like tea, water, infant formula, fruit juice, cow's milk, guimag (cow's milk with butter and flour), hashil (flour, water and sugar), or rice water with katik (kefir) or suzma (cottage cheese).
- Breastfeed frequently on demand at least 10–12 times in 24 hours, including 1 or 2 night feeds.
- Have your breastfeeding technique assessed by the health worker and follow any changes that he or she might suggest.
- Increase body contact with the baby, such as holding the baby in the hands, giving him or her a gentle hug or taking the baby to the bed where the mother sleeps.

From 4 to 6 months

Ideal feeding pattern
exclusive breastfeeding.

Give complementary foods two times a day *after* breastfeeding if the child:
- shows interest in semi-solid foods;
- is hungry after breastfeeding; or
- does not gain weight adequately.

Box 1. An example of a revised "food box" from Azerbaijan, March 1999

6–11 months of age

Porridge (semolina, rice, buckwheat, oat) + butter + milk (diluted 1:1)

Bread

Vegetable purée (potatoes, carrots, cabbage, onions)

Red meat, poultry, fish, liver, egg yolk

Katik, kefir, suzma

Fruit mash or juice (apple, mandarin, other seasonal fruits)

Do not give black tea

Use little if any salt and sugar

12–23 months of age

Give adequate servings of family foods or specially prepared foods, such as :

- rice, "pasta" or porridge (semolina, buckwheat, oatmeal, rice flour)
- vegetable purée (potatoes, carrots, beans, other seasonal vegetables)
- meat, including liver, poultry, fish, eggs
- katik, kefir, suzma
- bread
- fresh fruit (apples, other seasonal fruits)

Do not give black tea

Use little if any salt and sugar

24 months of age and above

Bread + cheese (brinza, shor, tuarog) or meat

Katik + (cottage) cheese + bread (or biscuits)

Fresh fruits or vegetables (carrots, tomatoes, cucumbers)

Cow's milk or kefir or katik

Do not give black tea

Use little salt and sugar

Counsel the mother about feeding problems

Suggest giving more frequent, on-demand, longer breastfeeding, day and night and gradually excluding other milk, foods and drinks

Give the child food in a separate plate or bowl and help the child to eat with own spoon

If the child is given black tea, replace the tea with breast-milk (< 6 months) or water or other liquids (> 6 months)

If the child's foods do not contain enough iron-rich sources:

- recommend increasing the amount of red meat and liver
- follow up any feeding problem in 5 days

Problem 2. Breastfeeding is being replaced or reduced too quickly.

Recommendations

- Breastfeed as often as the child wants.
- Give complementary foods after breastfeeding only if the child shows signs of hunger or if he or she does not gain adequate weight.

Problem 3. Child is being bottle-fed.

Recommendations

- Stop using bottles; give only breast-milk.
- If unavoidable, use home-prepared formula (1/4 cup cow's milk, 1/4 cup water, 1 teaspoon sugar or thin rice water + katik). Feed using cup and spoon.
- If unavoidable and if the family can afford it, use iron-supplemented infant formula prepared correctly. Feed using cup and spoon.

From 6 to 12 months

Ideal feeding pattern

Continue breastfeeding. Feed complementary foods three times a day if the child is breastfed, and five times a day if not breastfed. At each meal give adequate servings of, for example, vegetable mashes (potatoes and carrots); guimag; hashil with buckwheat, oatmeal or rice flour instead of wheat flour and reduced sugar; rice with katik or suzma; bread; and fruits such as apples and kiwi. Reduce the amounts of sugar and salt used. Avoid giving tea.

Problem 4. Complementary foods have not been started or foods that are not nutritionally adequate are given. In particular, the child's diet does not contain iron-rich foods.

Recommendation

- Give adequate servings of vegetable mashes (potatoes, carrots, beet, pumpkin, cauliflower, greens); or buckwheat, oatmeal or rice flour instead of wheat flour; or kefir or cottage cheese; or bread; or fruits; or egg/chicken/meat/liver/fish. Give within 30 minutes of cooking.

Problem 5. The child is being given too much sugar.

Recommendations

- Gradually reduce the amount of sugar used in food preparation.
- Stop giving the child candies, cakes and pastries.
- Avoid sweet drinks.

Problem 6. Salt is added to foods prepared for the child.

Recommendation

- Avoid adding salt to the child's food.

Problem 7. The child is being given black tea.

Recommendation

- Avoid using tea. Use breast-milk, plain water, fruit water or fruit juice instead.

Problem 8. The amount of food fed to the child is inadequate (frequency less than recommended or amount at each meal less than recommended for that age).

Recommendations

- Give one extra meal to the child. Gradually increase the number of meals to the recommended number.
- At each meal give the child one additional tablespoon till the child is ultimately consuming the recommended amount.

From 12 to 23 months

Ideal feeding pattern

Breastfeeding to be continued. The child should be eating the family diet plus extra feeds. Give family foods such as vermicelli, pilaff, vegetables (tomatoes, carrots), mashed vegetables (potatoes, carrots, pumpkin), meat, rice flour with katik or suzma, porridge with milk, bread, biscuits, fruit (apples, kiwi), cow's milk, kefir or other dairy products (suzma, gaymag, curd, cottage cheese). Feed at least five times a day. Reduce the amounts of sugar and salt used. Avoid giving tea.

Problem 9. The child is not yet being given family foods or foods are not nutritionally adequate.

Recommendation:

- Give the child vermicelli, pilaff, mashed vegetables (potatoes, carrots), meat, porridge with milk, bread, biscuits, fruit, kefir and legumes (peas, beans, green beans). Give within 30 minutes of cooking.

Problem 10. The child is being given inadequate amounts, i.e. meals less than five times a day or less than 300 ml per meal.

Recommendations

- Give one extra meal to the child. Slowly increase the number of meals until the child is eating five meals a day.
- Feed the child one extra tablespoon of food at each meal. Keep increasing the amount until the child is eating the advised amount at each meal.

Problem 11. The child refuses to eat.

Recommendations

- Give the child his or her favourite foods.
- Treat the child if ill.
- Play with the child while feeding, sing or use different ways to encourage the child to eat.
- Sit next to the child and patiently help with eating.